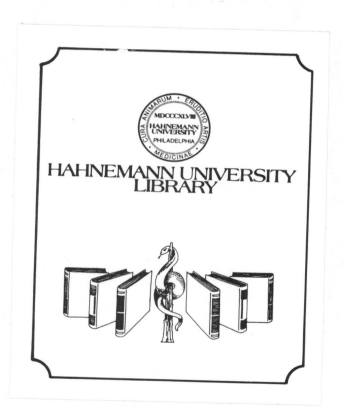

Comprehensive Manuals of Surgical Specialties

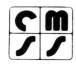

Richard H. Egdahl, editor

Walter Lawrence Jr., James P. Neifeld,
and Jose J. Terz

Manual of Soft-Tissue Tumor Surgery

Illustrated by Jane Hurd and Trudy Nicholson

Includes 248 Illustrations in Full Color, 19 Illustrations
in Black and White, and 43 Line Drawings.

Springer-Verlag
New York   Berlin   Heidelberg   Tokyo

SERIES EDITOR

Richard H. Egdahl, M.D., PH.D., Professor of Surgery, Boston University Medical Center, Boston, Massachusetts 02118, U.S.A.

AUTHORS

Walter Lawrence Jr., M.D., Professor and Chairman, Division of Surgical Oncology, and Director, Massey Cancer Center, Medical College of Virginia (Virginia Commonwealth University), P.O. Box 11, Richmond, Virginia 23298, U.S.A.

James P. Neifeld, M.D., Associate Professor, Division of Surgical Oncology, and Member, Massey Cancer Center, Medical College of Virginia (Virginia Commonwealth University), MCV Station, P.O. Box 11, Richmond, Virginia 23298, U.S.A.

Jose J. Terz, M.D., Director, Department of General Oncologic Surgery, City of Hope National Medical Center, 1500 East Duarte Road, Duarte, California 91010, U.S.A.

MEDICAL ILLUSTRATORS

Jane Hurd, 4002 Virginia Place, Bethesda, Maryland 20816
Trudy Nicholson, 7400 Arden Road, Cabin John, Maryland 20818

Library of Congress Cataloging in Publication Data
Lawrence, Walter, 1925–
    Manual of soft-tissue tumor surgery.

    Comprehensive manuals of surgical specialties

    Bibliography: p.
    Includes index.
    1. Sarcoma—Surgery—Addresses, essays, lectures.
I. Neifeld, James P.   II. Terz, Jose J.   III. Title.
IV. Series.   [DNLM: 1. Soft tissue neoplasms—Surgery—
Handbooks.   2. Sarcoma—Surgery—Handbooks.   WD 375
L424m]
RD651.L36   1983   616.99′4059   83–10605

Illustration Consultant: Fredric M. Harwin
Design and Layout by Caliber Design Planning, Inc.
Typeset by Kingsport Press, Kingsport, Tennessee
Color Separations by R. R. Donnelley & Sons Company, Crawfordsville, Indiana
Printed and Bound by R. R. Donnelley & Sons Company, Crawfordsville, Indiana
Printed in the United States of America.

9 8 7 6 5 4 3 2 1

ISBN   0–387–90843–9   Springer-Verlag   New York   Berlin   Heidelberg   Tokyo
ISBN   3–540–90843–9   Springer-Verlag   Berlin   Heidelberg   New York   Tokyo

Contents

Contents

Editor's Note

Comprehensive Manuals of Surgical Specialties is a series of surgical manuals designed to present current operative techniques and to explore various aspects of diagnosis and treatment. The series features a unique format with emphasis on large, detailed, full-color illustrations, schematic charts, and photographs to demonstrate integral steps in surgical procedures.

Each manual focuses on a specific region or topic and describes surgical anatomy, physiology, pathology, diagnosis, and operative treatment. Operative techniques and stratagems for dealing with surgically correctable disorders are described in detail. Illustrations are primarily depicted from the surgeon's viewpoint to enhance clarity and comprehension.

Other volumes in the series:

Published:

Manual of Endocrine Surgery
Manual of Burns
Manual of Surgery of the Gallbladder, Bile Ducts, and Exocrine Pancreas
Manual of Gynecologic Surgery
Manual of Urologic Surgery
Manual of Lower Gastrointestinal Surgery
Manual of Vascular Surgery, Volume I
Manual of Cardiac Surgery, Volume I
Manual of Cardiac Surgery, Volume II
Manual of Liver Surgery
Manual of Ambulatory Surgery
Manual of Pulmonary Surgery

In Preparation:

Manual of Vascular Surgery, Volume II
Manual of Orthopedic Surgery
Manual of Upper Gastrointestinal Surgery
Manual of Trauma Surgery
Manual of Sports Surgery
Manual of Aesthetic Plastic Surgery
Manual of Breast Surgery
Manual of Endocrine Surgery, 2nd edition

Richard H. Egdahl

Preface

The management of soft-tissue neoplasms has always had an aura of mystique due to the relative rarity of these lesions in comparison to the more common cancers occurring in man. There are many variations in technique of the operations employed for these tumors as well. In this volume we have illustrated our own personal preferences in approach to soft tissue sarcomas with the hope it will serve as a useful guide to the surgeon who is faced with one or more of these problems. None of the operations depicted in this manual are original with us but they are procedures and approaches we have found effective for the clinical management of this family of tumors.

In presenting this volume we wish to acknowledge our gratitude to our surgical teachers, our present and past associates in surgical oncology, our colleagues in the other oncologic disciplines, and our patients whose treatment is illustrated herein. We are indebted to Dr. Saul Kay, Professor of Pathology, and Dr. James Walsh, Associate Professor of Radiology, for providing the illustrations of histopathology and radiologic imaging in the early chapters. We particularly appreciate the superb artwork of our enthusiastic teammates, Trudy Nicholson and Jane Hurd, as their contribution is the crux of our endeavor.

Walter Lawrence Jr., M.D.
James P. Neifeld, M.D.
Jose J. Terz, M.D.

General Principles

I

Soft-Tissue Sarcomas: Etiology, Pathology, and Clinical Features

1

Soft-tissue sarcomas are uncommon cancers representing only 1% of all malignant neoplasms (excluding skin) in adults. The total number of soft-tissue sarcomas diagnosed each year in the United States is about 5000. In view of this, few surgeons have had enough experience with these lesions to appreciate the many variations in their clinical presentation or natural history. Also, owing to this limited incidence of sarcomas, few controlled clinical trials have been carried out to determine optimal treatment programs. Accordingly, many of the observations in this book will be based on our personal clinical experience, rather than thorough scientific study, but the available data will be reviewed.

Although soft-tissue sarcomas are relatively rare neoplasms, several large series have been reported which enable the clinician to develop some appreciation of the variations in the presentation and natural history of this family of tumors. In addition, collaborative investigations of potential prognostic features have been utilized to develop a useful clinical staging system for sarcomas. This first chapter will be concerned with a brief review of our knowledge of causation, variations in pathology, clinical presentation, and natural history of the various soft-tissue sarcomas. All of this will serve as an introduction to the practical aspects of evaluation and management to be described in subsequent chapters.

Etiology of Soft-Tissue Sarcomas

Although we have no definite information regarding causation, soft-tissue sarcomas have been etiologically related to several factors. These include various chemicals, radiation injury, chronic lymphedema, and a combination of these factors. The available information concerning these potential causes will be briefly reviewed.

Chemical Carcinogens

The development of sarcoma has been associated with exposure to several chemical substances many years prior to the clinical presentation. A series of reports from Sweden (6,37) and the United States (18,42,44) have suggested a causal relationship between exposure to phenoxy acids, or chlorophenols, and the subsequent development of soft-tissue sarcomas among workers in the railroad and chemical industries; the earlier reports are confirmed by two case-control studies (24,38). Although the latent period (time from first exposure) was relatively long, the duration of contact with phenoxy acids or chlorophenol was not well documented, nor was the exposure to other possible carcinogens in the environment. In addition, one patient was stated to have "potential exposure" (60) instead of direct exposure to these compounds. In one case-controlled study the increased risk of developing a soft-tissue sarcoma after exposure to phenoxy acids was 6.8 times greater than controls not previously exposed and 3.3 times greater following exposure to chlorophenols (24). Two American studies (62,96) from the chemical industry have been unable to confirm these results, but one of these studies has been criticized for not including all people exposed to chlorophenol. In addition, no deaths from soft-tissue sarcomas have been reported in three European studies of workers exposed to trichlorophenols or phenoxy acids in manufacturing (16). Phenoxy acids, which are derived from chlorophenols, release the by-product 2,3,7,8-tetrachlorodibenzo-p-dioxin (TCDD), which has been reported to produce soft-tissue sarcomas in rats (90). Increasing regulation has markedly decreased these impurities in the environment (16,21) and, consequently, may have markedly diminished the hazard of carcinogenic exposure to these compounds. It seems clear that further study of these and similar patient populations is required to further delineate the risk of soft-tissue sarcoma development following occupational exposure to phenoxy acids and the related chlorophenols.

Vinyl chloride gas, which is polymerized to form polyvinyl chloride (a widely used synthetic plastic), has been associated with the development of hepatic angiosarcomas in workers exposed for a long period of time (86). Although the incidence of angiosarcoma in this industrial setting could not be estimated, other histologic changes (including fibrosis and portal hypertension) were similar to the changes with chronic arsenical poisoning (71) and Thorotrast administration (89,91), following which angiosarcomas also occur. Recently, several cases of hepatic angiosarcoma have been associated with treatment with androgenic-anabolic steroids (26). In addition, the histologic changes in the liver following administration of these steroids are quite similar to the precursor lesions of hepatic angiosarcoma.

Although sarcomas have been shown to occur following viral exposure in various animal species, there is little reliable information regarding a potential viral cause of human sarcomas. Because a viral causation of sarcomas in man appears speculative at the present time, this aspect of carcinogenesis will not be reviewed.

Radiation as a Carcinogen

A number of sarcomas have subsequently developed in tissues receiving radiation for other neoplasms. Most postirradiation sarcomas arise in areas that have been subjected to relatively high doses of radiotherapy, but this is not always true. The dosage has ranged from 2000 to 10,000 rads (10,17,29,39, 41,59,66,87); many case reports do not state the exact amount of radiation administered.

Appropriate criteria for acceptance of prior radiation as an etiologic agent for sarcoma have been reported by Cahan (10). First, the sarcoma in question must be located in the previously irradiated area. This is usually fairly easy to determine by observation of skin changes associated with previous irradiation to the site. A second criterion is a prolonged latent period between the radiation therapy and the clinical appearance of the sarcoma. It is unusual to have a latent period of less than ten years for most radiation-induced sarcomas, although several cases of sarcoma after irradiation have been reported with shorter latent periods than this. A third criterion is, of course, the appearance of a different histologic type of cancer. If the histology of the neoplasm under consideration is the same as that of a previously treated cancer, it must be assumed that the second tumor is merely a recurrence of the initial process.

Many sarcomas have been reported following radiation treatments for either breast cancer or other malignant tumors. Although the incidence of postirradiation sarcoma is difficult to determine, it has been estimated to arise in 0.03% to 0.2% of breast cancer patients who received radiation (41,66). All types of sarcomas have been reported following radiation, including bone sarcomas (66). Osteosarcomas have been reported in many unusual locations, including the scapula and clavicle, following breast irradiation (41); they usually occur in older patients, whereas most nonradiation-induced osteosarcomas occur in teenagers and young adults. Fibrosarcomas are the most common soft-tissue sarcoma occurring after irradiation.

Sarcomas have been reported following radiation for gynecologic cancer (67), head and neck cancer (17), skin cancer, lymphoma, and benign conditions such as thymic enlargement, endometriosis, and even tuberculosis (7). The average latent interval has been about 11 years, and the symptoms leading to diagnosis include the onset of pain or swelling in the previously irradiated area. Examination will often reveal postirradiation changes, including hyperpigmentation, telangiectasias, fibrosis, and ulceration. Treatment of the sarcoma is surgical, and most radiation-induced extremity sarcomas require amputation. Nevertheless, the overall prognosis is poor, with few long-term, disease-free survivors.

An uncommon sarcoma that occurs after irradiation but is associated with chronic lymphedema is lymphangiosarcoma (49,58,61,72,79,82,95). Stewart and Treves (82) first described lymphangiosarcoma developing in lymphedematous arms following mastectomy for carcinoma of the breast in 1948. Since that time many reports have appeared. The common denominator in these patients has been significant chronic lymphedema following surgery; in the updated series from the Memorial Sloan-Kettering Cancer Center (79), 22 of 34 patients developing lymphangiosarcoma following mastectomy had received postoperative radiotherapy. The sarcomas appeared from 7 to 23 years following mastectomy and were outside the radiated field in most instances. The role of radiation in the causation of this form of sarcoma is not that of a direct carcinogen but is related to its contribution to the arm edema after axillary dissection and radiation to the axillary area. The benign counterpart to lymphangiosarcoma, lymphangioma circumscriptum, has also been reported following mastectomy and radiation therapy (69) but is less common than lymphangiosarcoma.

Other Causes

Most sarcomas have no prior radiation and no chemical agents or viral agents that can be implicated in their causation. In some instances, such as von Recklinghausen's disease, inherited factors play a role. However, for most patients with sarcoma, we have no real clue regarding causation. Possibly environmental exposure to carcinogens, either chemical or viral, is important, but there is no evidence for any major etiologic factors at the present time.

FIG. 1-1. These patients demonstrate the variable gross presentation of soft-tissue sarcomas. They frequently present as masses within muscle compartments (**A**) but may occur in the subcutaneous plane outside the fascial layers (**B**). The malignant hemangiopericytoma of the buttock in **C** is a primary process in the skin itself, as is the classic dermatofibrosarcoma protuberans shown in **D**.

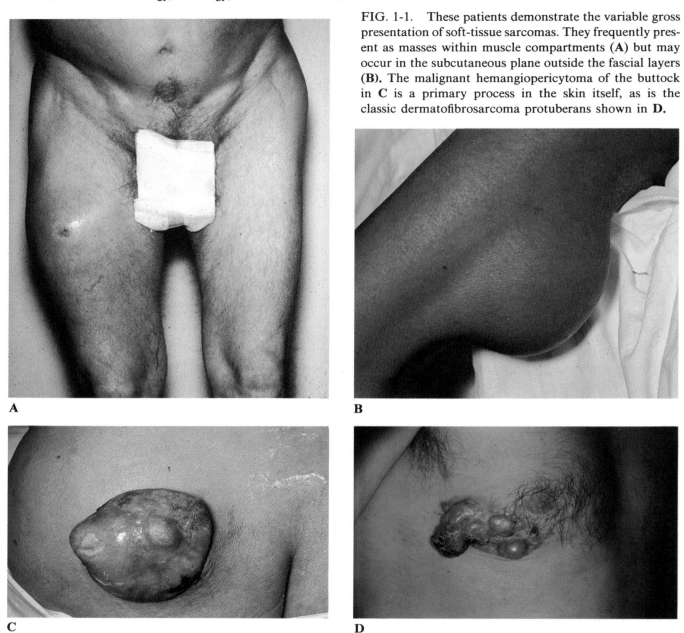

A

B

C

D

Clinical Presentation of Soft-Tissue Sarcoma

This group of malignant neoplasms has been described in virtually all anatomic locations, although in adults there is a preponderance of lesions in areas where there is a bulk of mesodermal tissue (e.g., extremities, particularly the thigh). Also, variations in location and predominant age group seem to occur with differing histologic classifications (such as distal extremity locations in young adults with synovial sarcoma). Less often the clinical presentation may be a dermal nodule or a mass within a major body cavity (such as those sarcomas arising from the mesoderm of the gastrointestinal tract or retroperitoneum). However, the usual clinical presentation is that of a nonspecific solid mass in the subcutaneous or deeper tissues (Fig. 1-1). It may be brought to attention by its physical size, discomfort, or more often a recent change in size of a

6

mass noted by the otherwise asymptomatic patient. The heterogeneous nature of the possible clinical presentations is further compounded by the variations in histology. Although the differing histologic types, and presumed histogenetic origins, may prove to be of less importance than other features of these sarcomas (such as size, anatomic location, histologic differentiation), it is most convenient to approach a detailed description of these sarcomas with the standard histologic classifications. These are based on the presumed cell origin of the individual neoplasms.

Patterns of Spread of Soft-Tissue Sarcomas

Soft-tissue sarcomas spread via direct local invasion, lymphatics, and hematogenous dissemination. Locally these tumors spread within tissue planes and along nerve sheaths, vessels, and fascial compartments. Thus, patients undergoing limited local resections of sarcomas have a high likelihood of local recurrence, whereas patients who undergo aggressive wide resections, to include an adequate normal tissue plane in all directions around the tumor, have a low incidence of local recurrence (see Chapter 3).

The incidence of metastatic soft-tissue sarcoma depends upon the primary site, histology, and most importantly the degree of differentiation. Regional lymph nodes are only rarely involved in patients undergoing treatment for soft-tissue sarcoma, and lymph node involvement tends to occur mainly with synovial sarcomas and malignant fibrous histiocytomas. A major problem with most reports of lymphatic metastasis is that the incidence often includes autopsy as well as clinical data; the nodal metastases listed may be regional or distant, and almost invariably the lymphatic spread is associated with widespread metastatic disease. Weingrad and Rosenberg (92) reviewed the situation from the standpoint of regional lymph node dissection for adults with soft-tissue sarcoma. Although some specific sarcomas in adults seem to have a higher frequency of nodal metastasis than others, there is little evidence that treatment of regional nodes by dissection has a major affect on prognosis. In the absence of clinically apparent nodal metastases, it is clear that prophylactic lymph node dissection is not indicated in the management of adult patients with soft-tissue sarcomas. Fortunately lymphatics are rarely an initial route of regional spread for the adult sarcoma population.

Few studies have examined the incidence of metastatic disease in patients at the time of initial presentation of a clinically localized soft-tissue sarcoma. The major site of distant hematogenous metastasis is the lungs, with other sites, particularly the liver, much less frequent. This is the basis for the effectiveness of pulmonary resection for selected patients (see Chapter 12). Fortunately, most soft-tissue sarcomas are confined to the anatomic area of the primary site at initial clinical presentation (see Chapter 2).

Posttreatment evaluation of patients with soft-tissue sarcoma is required to determine the natural history of this family of tumors. Over 80% of all treatment failures occur within the first two years, and most in the first year following treatment. Sarcomas that recur later than this tend to be the better differentiated, more slow-growing tumors, such as well-differentiated fibrosarcomas and dermatofibrosarcoma protuberans. The site of recurrence is usually the primary site and/or pulmonary metastases. Thus the clinical strategy for following patients after treatment of a primary sarcoma should include clinical examination fairly frequently during the first two years along with periodic chest x-rays; the value of routine postoperative whole-lung tomography or computed tomography is yet to be determined. As recurrences are fairly uncommon more than two years following initial surgery, the routine clinical examinations and chest x-rays can then be performed less frequently.

Classification of Sarcomas

The great majority of soft-tissue sarcomas are thought to arise from the primitive mesoderm. Of the three primitive germ cell layers (i.e., endoderm, mesoderm, ectoderm), the ectoderm gives rise to neurofibrosarcomas (or malignant neurilemmomas), whereas the mesoderm is thought to give rise to most other sarcomas (Table 1-1). Most sarcomas have benign neoplastic counterparts; for example, fat cells may give rise to lipomas or liposarcomas, fibroblasts may give rise to fibromas as well as fibrosarcomas, and smooth muscle may give rise to leiomyomas as well as leiomyosarcomas. Some individual sarcomas are difficult to classify, and several of the sarcomas have a controversial cell of origin: the alveolar soft-part sarcoma, malignant fibrous histiocytoma, and epithelioid sarcoma have not been well classified as to the cell of origin although they are clearly defined pathologic entities.

Most pathologic diagnoses, from the standpoint of classification, have been made using conventional light microscopy. The addition of electron microscopy has refined diagnosis, particularly in terms of the presumed cell of origin. Well-differentiated sarcomas may be difficult to distinguish from benign neoplasms but they are conveniently classified as to probable mesodermal cell of origin. Undifferentiated sarcomas may be impossible to classify histogenetically, even with the aid of the electron microscope.

Although histogenetic classification has been the major focus of both pathologists and clinicians over the years, the clinical behavior, response to treatment, and prognosis appear to have a stronger correlation with the degree of differentiation. The "grade" of the sarcoma, and the AJC staging system that incorporates this characteristic, will be reviewed from its clinical aspects in Chapter 2. For this initial discussion of histology, presentation, and natural history, the conventional histologic classification of sarcomas will be employed.

Table 1-1. Cell of Origin of Soft-Tissue Sarcomas

Germ cell layer	Normal cell	Sarcoma
Ectoderm	Nerve cell sheath	Neurofibrosarcoma
		Alveolar soft-part sarcoma (?)
Mesoderm	Adipose cell	Liposarcoma
	Fibroblast	Fibrosarcoma
		Dermatofibrosarcoma problems
		Malignant fibrous histiocytoma (?)
	Smooth muscle	Leiomyosarcoma
	Skeletal muscle	Rhabdomyosarcoma
	Tendosynovial cell	Synovial sarcoma
		Epithelioid sarcoma (?)
		Malignant giant cell tumor
	Blood vessel	Angiosarcoma
		Hemangiopericytoma
		Lymphangiosarcoma
		Kaposi's sarcoma
	Miscellaneous	Malignant mesenchymoma
		Malignant granular cell tumor

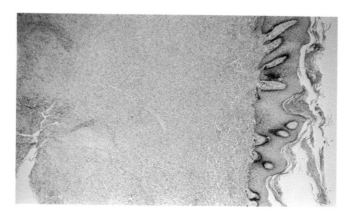

FIG. 1-2. Dermatofibroma. The tumor occupies the dermis and is covered by hyperplastic epidermis. Termed also benign fibrous histiocytoma.

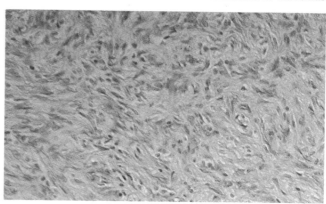

FIG. 1-3. Higher-power view of dermatofibroma. Note storiform or whirligig pattern of uniform, nonanaplastic spindle nuclei.

Fibrous Tissue

Tumors of fibrous tissue origin range from the benign dermatofibroma (Figs. 1-2, 1-3) to fibrosarcomas of varying degrees of differentiation (Figs. 1-4 to 1-8). Dermatofibromas (benign fibrous histiocytomas) are common tumors which are never malignant. They arise from fibroblasts and usually present as a nodule in the dermis.

Fibrosarcomas are malignant tumors which also arise from fibroblasts; they range from very well-differentiated tumors, which rarely metastasize, to poorly differentiated, bizarre tumors with a paucity of collagen and frequent evidence of hematogenous metastasis. The great majority of fibrosarcomas arise on the extremities (32), and they are most commonly seen in the fifth to seventh decade of life. As in most categories of sarcoma, survival data have a direct correlation with the degree of histologic differentiation (70).

A variant of well-differentiated fibrosarcoma, the dermatofibrosarcoma protuberans (64) is a relatively rare dermal tumor with a marked propensity to recur at the local site after surgical excision, which is often narrowly accomplished owing to the deceivingly innocuous clinical presentation. It first appears as a single dermal nodule, either pink or blue in color, is freely mobile on the underlying tissues, and increases in size at a slow rate. After a period of time, or after limited excision, satellite nodules may appear and the tumor

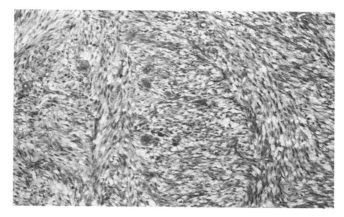

FIG. 1-4. Fibrosarcoma of ankle (well differentiated). Note herringbone pattern of uniform spindle cells.

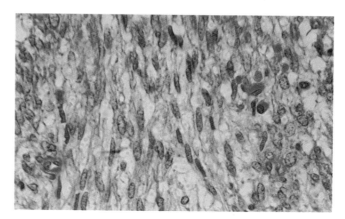

FIG. 1-5. Higher-power view of fibrosarcoma to show well-polarized spindle cells with bland nuclei.

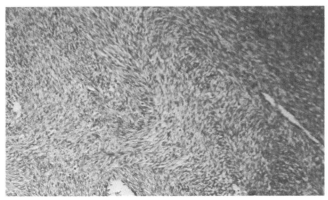

FIG. 1-6. Fibrosarcoma (moderate differentiation). The tumor is more cellular than in well-differentiated forms. Nuclei are crowed but still well polarized.

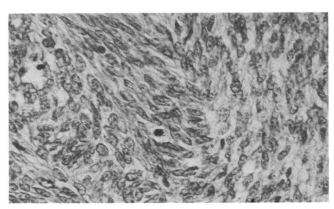

FIG. 1-7. Higher-power view of fibrosarcoma to show some degree of anaplasia with a mitotic figure in center.

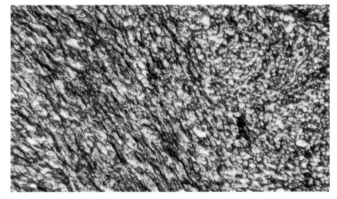

FIG. 1-8. A reticulin stain shows individual-cell wrapping of reticulin fibers.

begins to appear more exophytic. The nodules may coalesce and repeated trauma may lead to ulceration and bleeding. This lesion rarely metastasizes but progressive local invasion may produce severe disability and possibly death.

Malignant fibrous histiocytomas are sarcomas of uncertain histogenesis which have been associated with a poor prognosis, appearing to have both histiocytic and fibroblastic features (43,85) (Figs. 1-9 to 1-11). Since its first description in 1961, the malignant fibrous histiocytoma has been more and more commonly diagnosed (45,48,93); currently, it is one of the most frequently diagnosed soft-tissue sarcomas in adults (34). Many previously unclassified tumors or pleomorphic variants of other sarcomas have been reclassified now as malignant fibrous histiocytomas. Numerous histologic variants of this lesion have been described (fibrous, giant cell, myxoid, and inflammatory), but in larger series, the prognosis is no different among these various subtypes. Malignant fibrous histiocytomas may metastasize hematogenously (usually to the lungs) or lymphatically; of all the soft-tissue sarcomas in adults, they have the highest incidence of lymph node metastases. Anatomic location is a major factor in prognosis; superficial lesions have a better prognosis than deeper ones, and retroperitoneal sites have a poor prognosis.

Adipose Tissue

Tumors that arise from fat also range from benign to highly malignant sarcomas that metastasize to distant sites, usually the lungs. Benign fatty tumors,

10

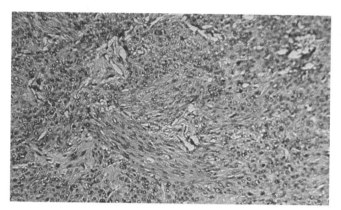

FIG. 1-9. Malignant fibrous histiocytoma. The malignant cells act as facultative fibroblasts imparting a storiform pattern to parts of the tumor.

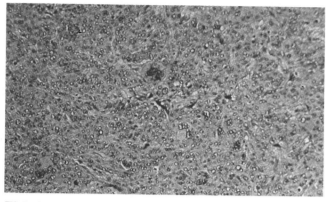

FIG. 1-10. Another field of the malignant fibrous histiocytoma showing scattered, extremely bizarre, multinucleated cells.

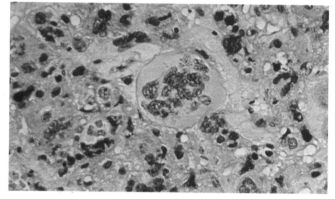

FIG. 1-11. A high-power view of the multinucleated cell of malignant fibrous histiocytoma. Intracytoplasmic fat is scanty and not nearly as abundant as in the multinucleated lipoblast of liposarcoma.

lipomas, are usually encapsulated, soft, slow-growing or static over a long period of time, and have the histologic appearance of normal fat tissue when removed by simple local excision. A rare benign tumor in infants and children, the lipoblastoma, is a lobulated encapsulated tumor which is also treated adequately by simple enucleation (84).

Liposarcomas range from the well-differentiated and myxoid varieties to the highly undifferentiated pleomorphic variant (Figs. 1-12 to 1-16). In most circumstances these tumors present as a relatively "pure" form, but it is not unusual to find more than one histologic pattern or a change in histologic pattern with recurrence or metastasis. In contrast to most sarcomas, which usually arise in the extremities, liposarcomas often arise in the retroperitoneum as well (8,47). In fact, the most frequent sarcoma in this site is a liposarcoma. Although extremity liposarcomas have a generally good prognosis after operative treatment (12,23,50,63), retroperitoneal liposarcomas have a poor prognosis (15) for the anatomic reasons discussed in Chapter 7.

Interestingly, recurrences of liposarcomas often tend to be more undifferentiated than the primary lesion. This histologic pattern of recurrence may cause diagnostic difficulties (78); and because the recurrent tumor may appear to be another histologic type, it tends to support the concept that most soft-tissue sarcomas are derived from a pluripotential stem cell (35).

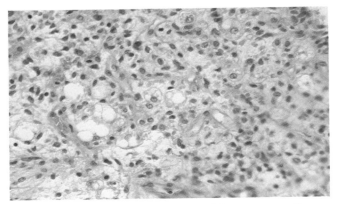

FIG. 1-12. Myxoid liposarcoma. The tumor cells are crowded and poorly differentiated but show evidence of lipid production, as evidenced by intracytoplasmic vacuoles.

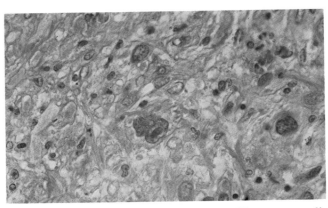

FIG. 1-13. Pleomorphic liposarcoma. The tumor cells show little resemblance to lipoblasts, are bizarre and multinucleated.

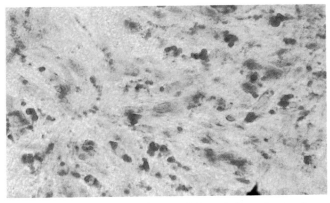

FIG. 1-14. A fat stain shows pink staining of cytoplasm diagnostic of lipid. Same case as Figure 1-13.

FIG. 1-15. Liposarcoma (round cell or adenoid type). Lipoblastic activity is seen on the left, and round dedifferentiated small tumor cells are seen on the right.

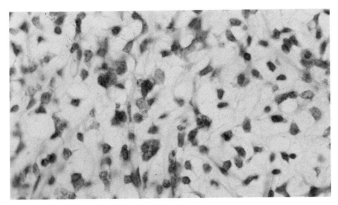

FIG. 1-16. High-power view of liposarcoma to show darkly staining round cells with irregular hyperchromatic nuclei.

Skeletal Muscle

Benign skeletal muscle tumors, rhabdomyomas (Figs. 1-17 and 1-18), are rare and most commonly located in the head and neck (20). They do not recur after complete local excision.

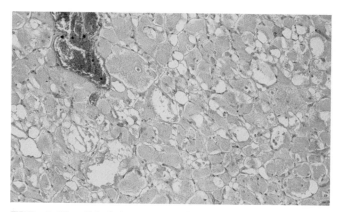

FIG. 1-17. Rhabdomyoma of floor of mouth. This is a tumor made up of mature myoblasts. The cells vary in size but there are no anaplastic nuclei.

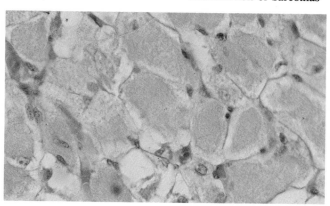

FIG. 1-18. High-power view reveals details of rhabdomyoblasts. The cytoplasm shows distinct matchsticklike fibrils simulating the cross striations of normal skeletal muscle.

Malignant skeletal muscle tumors, the rhabdomyosarcomas (Figs. 1-19 to 1-24), are the most common childhood soft-tissue sarcoma as well as being one of the more common adult soft-tissue sarcomas (5,46,53,81). The histologic rhabdomyosarcoma subtypes have been embryonal, alveolar, and pleomorphic, but terminology for childhood rhabdomyosarcoma has been changing as a result of the uniform pathologic classification of the large group study (IRS) described in Chapter 13. The embryonal category is the most favorable, while alveolar and other unfavorable histologic categories are associated with more frequent metastases and treatment failure. Sarcoma botryoides, which is seen in children, is a variant of embryonal rhabdomyosarcoma in the vagina, bladder, or nasophyaryngeal area and is characterized by being grossly polypoid and grapelike. The prognosis of rhabdomyosarcoma in children correlates with both primary site and the histologic category. The degree of differentiation (or "grade") is not a good prognostic indicator for rhabdomyosarcoma since virtually all these lesions are poorly differentiated.

Rhabdomyosarcomas in adults are commonly of the pleomorphic variety. They are most commonly located on the extremities (about 80%), in contrast to the distribution noted in children (Chapter 13), and the most common age group is the fifth to sixth decade. Prognosis tends to be poor in comparison

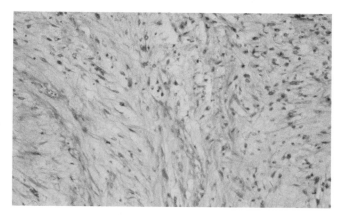

FIG. 1-19. Embryonal rhabdomyosarcoma. The tumor cells are elongated and spindly and set in a loose myxoid matrix.

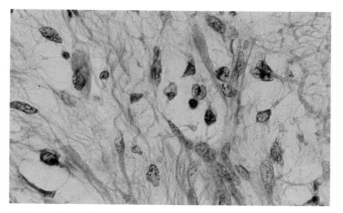

FIG. 1-20. High power to show undifferentiated cells with fibrillar tapering cytoplasm. Cross striations are generally indistinct and difficult to find.

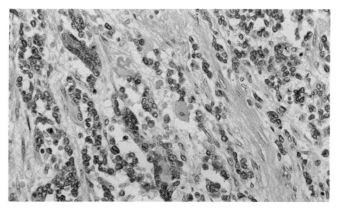

FIG. 1-21. Alveolar rhabdomyosarcoma. There is a vague glandular pattern with highly anaplastic nuclei. The rhabdomyoblast is identified by the large cell with almost homogeneous pink cytoplasm.

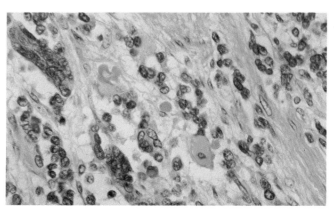

FIG. 1-22. High power to show details of tumor cells. The identifiable rhabdomyoblasts are in the center of the field.

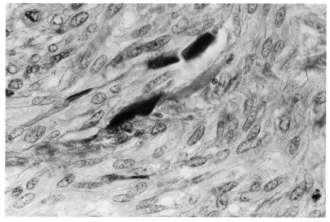

FIG. 1-23. Pleomorphic rhabdomyosarcoma. The tumor cells show undifferentiation with strap cell formation and hyperchromatic, extremely bizarre nuclei.

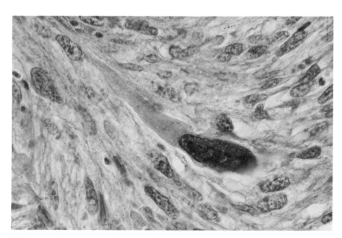

FIG. 1-24. Another field to show an elongated strap cell with suggestive cross striation.

with most of the other common sarcomas due to the undifferentiated nature of the tumor. The lungs are the major metastatic site.

Smooth Muscle

Tumors of smooth muscle range from the benign leiomyoma to malignant leiomyosarcoma (Figs. 1-25, 1-26). Both often arise in the wall of the gastrointestinal tract. Although benign leiomyomas may present as an asymptomatic abdominal mass, more commonly gastrointestinal bleeding or intestinal obstruction will be the presenting symptom. Other sites include the retroperitoneal area, skin and subcutaneous tissues, and rarely major veins.

Leiomyosarcomas are the most common sarcoma arising from the gastrointestinal tract, with stomach and small bowel sites being the most frequent (2,4,14,19,52,76,94). These tumors may grow to a very large size prior to the onset of symptoms; occasionally hemorrhage into the tumor with concomitant rapid increase in size may be the initial presentation. Leiomyosarcoma may be difficult to differentiate from leiomyoma on pathologic study; counting the number of mitoses per high-power field is the usual method for determining malignancy, but clinical behavior (i.e., leiomyosarcomas will invade adjacent tissues and metastasize whereas leiomyomas will not) is definitive. For leiomyo-

14

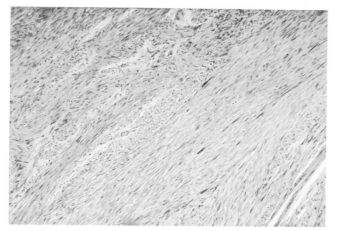

FIG. 1-25. Leiomyosarcoma. Palisaded well-differentiated smooth muscle cells are shown. There is little anaplasia of nuclei.

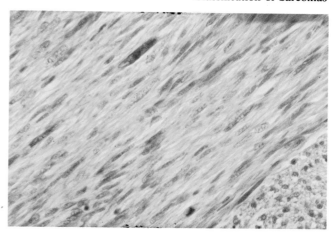

FIG. 1-26. High-power view of leiomyosarcoma to show blunted nuclear ends. Bizarre nucleus is seen on top, and atypical mitosis is seen on bottom.

sarcomas that originate in the bowel, with its portal venous drainage, distant metastases tend to be hepatic rather than pulmonary. Long-term survival of patients with gastrointestinal leiomyosarcomas is generally in the range of 30%–40%; patients with a long duration of symptoms, a small tumor, and no lymphatic metastases tend to have a better prognosis. Retroperitoneal leiomyosarcomas are associated with a much poorer prognosis (see Chapter 7).

Leiomyosarcomas arising in the skin or subcutaneous tissue are unusual tumors with a much better prognosis than those in either retroperitoneal or gastrointestinal primary sites (28). Cutaneous leiomyosarcomas rarely metastasize; subcutaneous leiomyosarcomas may recur and metastasize and should be treated more aggressively than the cutaneous lesions.

Schwann Cell Sheath

Most tumors arising from nerve cell sheaths are benign; many names have been applied, including schwannoma, neurilemmoma, and neurofibroma (Figs. 1-27, 1-28). They are especially common in patients with von Recklinghausen's disease. Neoplasms of nerve cell sheaths are virtually never malignant when located centrally, i.e., in the spinal cord, but may become malignant elsewhere in the body.

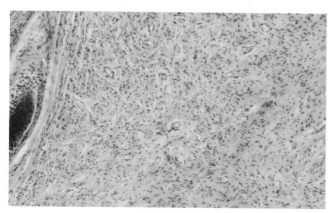

FIG. 1-27. Neurofibroma within the dermis of a patient with von Recklinghausen's disease. Note irregular whorls of spindled Schwann cells. Hair follicle on left.

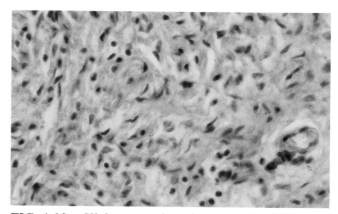

FIG. 1-28. High-power view shows details of Schwann cells, which are bland and separated by a fibrillar eosinophilic stroma.

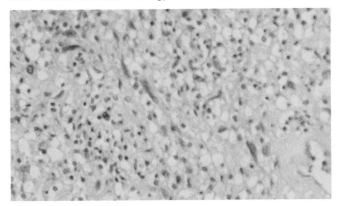

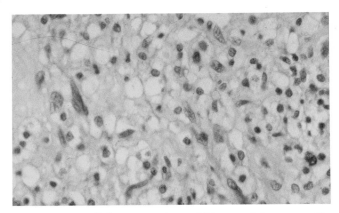

FIG. 1-29.   Malignant schwannoma. The tumor cells are irregularly scattered within the stroma, with evidence of crowding. Isolated bizarre elements are noted.

FIG. 1-30.   High-power view of bizarre Schwann cells.

Malignant nerve cell sheath tumors (malignant Schwannoma, malignant neurilemmoma, neurofibrosarcoma) are most commonly found on the extremities (25,33,80,83,88). They tend to be poorly differentiated tumors with their origin usually from the sheath surrounding small nerves, rather than from major nerves. Due to the undifferentiated nature of these lesions, prognosis tends to be poor (Figs. 1-29, 1-30). They rarely metastasize to lymph nodes, but hematogenous metastasis, primarily pulmonary, is common.

Patients with disseminated neurofibromatosis (von Recklinghausen's disease) with a sarcoma tend to have a slightly different clinical setting and course than patients with neurofibrosarcomas arising de novo. The von Recklinghausen patients tend to be somewhat younger at the time of sarcoma diagnosis, have tumor more often centrally located (such as the trunk or neck), and have a somewhat worse prognosis than patients with spontaneously arising neurofibrosarcomas. This poorer prognosis may be related to the more frequent central location of the primary tumor rather than any inherent difference in the sarcomas arising in the two patient groups.

Synovial Tissues

Most neoplasms arising from synovium are malignant; these are termed synovial sarcoma or tendosynovial sarcoma (9,11,30,36,77). Interestingly, this sarcoma is rarely associated with the synovium of joint spaces, despite its name. Most synovial sarcomas arise from aponeurotic fascia, tendon, tendon sheath, or synovial bursa. The great majority of these tumors arise distally in the extremities, and they have been classified into two major histopathologic forms: the biphasic synovial sarcoma, which has a better prognosis, and the monophasic synovial sarcoma, with a somewhat worse prognosis (Figs. 1-31 to 1-34).

Synovial sarcomas tend to be poorly differentiated and have a higher rate of local recurrence and distant metastases after surgical treatment than most sarcomas. The incidence of regional lymph node metastases is relatively high (15%–20%), and few patients with lymph node metastases will be cured despite regional lymphadenectomy. Distant spread tends to be to the lungs, and the approach to treatment of pulmonary metastases is similar to that used for other sarcomas (Chapter 12).

Vascular Endothelium

Tumors arising from vascular endothelium range from the benign juvenile hemangioendothelioma and hemangioma to the malignant hemangiopericy-

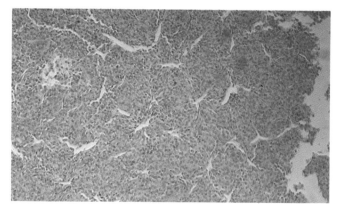

FIG. 1-31. The monophasic synovial sarcoma reveals only the spindle element of the tumor, with often a striking resemblance to hemangiopericytoma due to the perivascular arrangement of the spindled tumor cells.

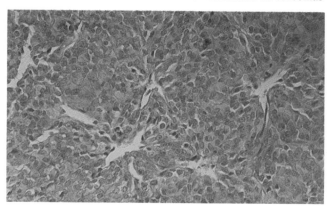

FIG. 1-32. A high-power view illustrates the crowded spindle elements encircling vascular spaces.

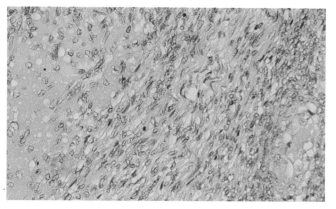

FIG. 1-33. Synovial sarcoma, biphasic type. The spindle fibroblastic pattern is predominant, with an epithelial glandlike structure in lower right.

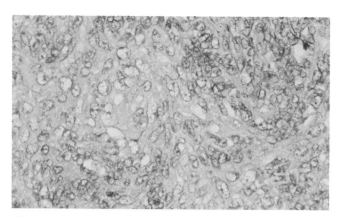

FIG. 1-34. Synovial sarcoma showing epithelial pattern. Same case as Figure 1-33.

toma, malignant hemangioendothelioma (angiosarcoma), and lymphangiosarcoma (discussed earlier).

Angiosarcomas most commonly arise on the scalp, face, breast, or extremities but they are relatively rare lesions (13,54). Small tumor size, distal location, and less pleomorphism on histologic examination are favorable prognostic features, but the overall prognosis is poor for angiosarcoma (Figs. 1-35, 1-36). Lymphatic and hematogenous spread is reported to be frequent.

Hemangiopericytomas are thought to arise from the capillary pericytes of Zimmermann, cells that spiral around the capillaries and postcapillary venules. Tumors with very few mitoses may follow a malignant course (Figs. 1-37,1-38); about half of all hemangiopericytomas are malignant. Although the short-term prognosis is good, significant numbers of patients will develop local recurrence and die after five years (31,57).

Kaposi's sarcoma (idiopathic multiple hemorrhagic sarcoma) (Fig. 1-39) is another variant of angiosarcoma with a unique clinical presentation. It usually presents as a bluish macule on the skin, but the diagnosis is rarely made until there are multiple nodules and lymphedema. It has a very similar gross and microscopic presentation to lymphangiosarcoma, arising in an extremity that is chronically edematous. When lymphangiosarcoma develops in a chronically edematous arm after radical mastectomy, it has been called the Stewart-Treves syndrome.

17

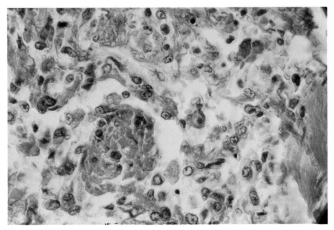

FIG. 1-35. Malignant hemangioendothelioma (angiosarcoma). Vascular spaces are lined by anaplastic endothelial cells.

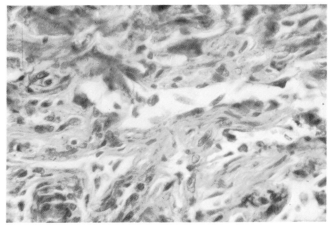

FIG. 1-36. Another area of tumor in Figure 1-35. The malignant endothelial cells are flattened and elongated but distinctly atypical.

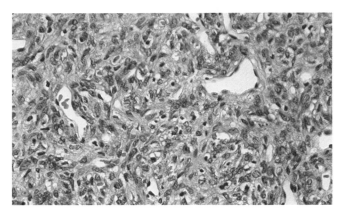

FIG. 1-37. Hemangiopericytoma. Vascular spaces are surrounded by spindled pericytes.

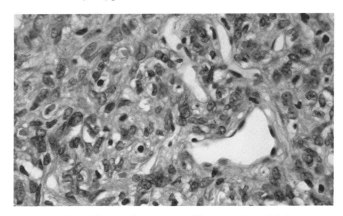

FIG. 1-38. The pericytes are illustrated at high power and are clearly outside the variously sized vascular spaces.

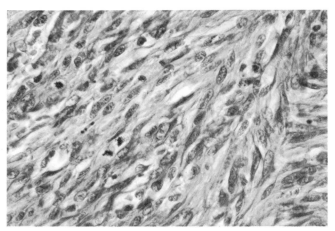

FIG. 1-39. Kaposi's sarcoma. Malignant spindle cells with vascular slits.

Miscellaneous Tumors

Other less common sarcomas have been described that are recognized as entities, but the histogenesis of these lesions is uncertain. The alveolar soft-part sarcoma (Figs. 1-40, 1-41) is such a tumor of uncertain histogenesis, but recently it has been related by some to the Schwann cell (22,56). This sarcoma occurs most often in young adults, usually arising in the extremities (51). It tends

18

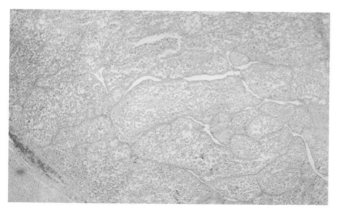

FIG. 1-40. Alveolar soft-part sarcoma. The organoid pattern of granular cells is emphasized.

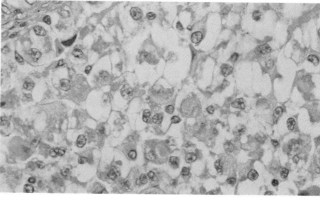

FIG. 1-41. High-power view shows details of granular cells.

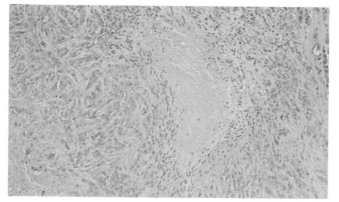

FIG. 1-42. Epithelioid sarcoma. A granulomatous pattern showing central necrosis surrounded by palisaded tumor cells. This tumor is considered by some to be a variant of synovial sarcoma.

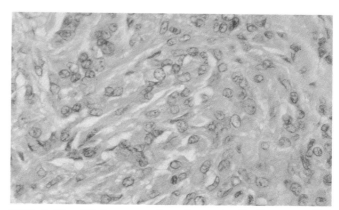

FIG. 1-43. High-power view shows detail of tumor cells, irregularly dispersed and crowded with vesicular nuclei.

to be slow-growing, with local recurrence documented in some patients more than ten years following resection.

Epithelioid sarcomas (Figs. 1-42, 1-43) are rare tumors, and they usually arise distally on an extremity (3,68). Histogenesis is unclear but some have attributed this tumor to synovial (65) or Schwann cells. These sarcomas tend to have a high incidence of lymph node metastases and vascular invasion on histologic examination. They may recur early but often have a prolonged course, despite their ultimately high rate of treatment failure.

Prognostic Criteria

Numerous factors have been evaluated as prognostic criteria affecting the clinical course of patients with soft-tissue sarcomas. These include primary site, tumor size, degree of differentiation, histologic type, and age.

Site: The primary site of soft-tissue sarcomas is of paramount importance in terms of both treatment strategy and prognosis. The more proximal the tumor is on the extremity, the worse the prognosis. Usually distal extremity lesions can be treated more easily than proximal lesions. Also, such treatment may be undertaken at an earlier stage, because distal lesions are less likely to be large than tumors located more proximally. For example, a small mass is much more likely to be detected distally on an extremity than if it is located deep in the quadriceps musculature or the buttock. Other anatomic sites pre-

19

Table 1-2. Tumor Size Correlated with Survival

Institution	Five-year survival	
	<5 cm	>5 cm
Roswell Park Memorial Institute (1)	57%	40%
Memorial Sloan-Kettering Cancer Center (75)	63%	46%

Table 1-3. Degree of Differentiation Correlated with Survival (75)

Size	Five-year survival	
	Low-grade tumor	High-grade tumor
<5 cm	88%	63%
>5 cm	58%	33%

clude the wide operative margins that are required to avoid recurrence; retroperitoneal, pelvic, trunk, and head and neck sites fit this category.

Size: The size of soft-tissue sarcomas will affect prognosis. A major criterion in the recently developed clinical staging system for soft-tissue sarcomas concerns tumor size (see Chapter 2). Patients presenting with sarcomas smaller than 5 cm have a superior prognosis compared with patients with tumors greater than 5 cm in size. Two large reviews demonstrate this relationship (Table 1-2). Several reasons could explain this decreasing prognosis with increasing tumor size. For example, large sarcomas are more likely to have neurovascular or bone involvement than are small tumors. Larger tumors are more difficult to treat locally from the standpoint of achieving adequate margins. Thus, for soft-tissue sarcomas, as for most other cancers, early diagnosis remains an important factor in improving prognosis.

Degree of differentiation: The most important prognostic variable is probably the degree of differentiation of the sarcoma (73). Table 1-3 shows how the prognosis varies according to degree of differentiation; patients with well-differentiated tumors do reasonably well, whereas patients with poorly differentiated tumors have less desirable disease-free survival statistics. These data have led to the addition of tumor grade to the AJC staging system for sarcomas, the T(umor) N(ode) M(etastasis) system (Chapter 2). Patients with high-grade sarcomas have a higher incidence of both local and distant failure than low-grade sarcomas. In addition, it has been shown that patients with recurrent sarcoma are more likely to have a tumor that is less well differentiated than was the primary tumor.

Histology: It has long been reported that the histology of the primary tumor is an important prognostic variable (74). Table 1-4 shows overall survival data for soft-tissue sarcoma patients correlated with histologic categories. In general, patients with rhabdomyosarcomas and synovial sarcomas have a worse prognosis than those with fibrosarcomas and liposarcomas. However, when one looks at the degree of differentiation of the primary tumor, histologic

Table 1-4. Histology of Soft-Tissue Sarcomas Correlated with Five-Year Survival (Adults)

Institution	Fibro-sarcoma	Leiomyo-sarcoma	Lipo-sarcoma	Neuro-fibro-sarcoma	Rhabdo-myo-sarcoma	Malignant fibrous histio-cytoma	Synovial sarcoma
UCLA (40)	60%	23%	78%		10%		60%
RPMI (1)	50	41	61	37%	31	67%	34
MCV (27)	82	60	78		29		
Göteberg (55)	80	50	82			40	50
MSKCC (75)	70		56	40	48		45

UCLA = University of California, Los Angeles; RPMI = Roswell Park Memorial Institute; MCV = Medical College of Virginia; Göteberg = University of Göteberg; MSKCC = Memorial Sloan-Kettering Cancer Center.

category seems to play a secondary role. Well-differentiated fibrosarcomas have the same prognosis as well-differentiated tumors with other histology, but most rhabdomyosarcomas, synovial sarcomas, and angiosarcomas tend to be poorly differentiated. Thus the histologic type may be more useful in suggesting the degree of differentiation than in determining prognosis by itself.

Age: Age does not appear to play a major role in determining prognosis in patients with soft-tissue sarcomas. Some studies suggest that patients with fibrosarcoma who are extremely young have a better prognosis than those who are older. This is not necessarily true within the pediatric group. However, when results of all sarcomas in the pediatric age group are compared with results of sarcomas in patients over 20 years of age, it is clear that children with fibrosarcomas and liposarcomas have a much better prognosis than adults. Rhabdomyosarcomas in childhood do seem to behave and respond quite differently than adult rhabdomyosarcomas, the children being much more responsive to different therapies. Most other sarcomas in childhood appear fairly similar to those in adults (see Chapter 13).

Comment

This background information on soft-tissue sarcomas illustrates the wide variation in clinical presentation, pathology, and natural history of these lesions. It clearly demonstrates the need for multiple variations in the management approach. Operative management remains a major consideration for therapy despite these differences, however, and this will be the primary focus of this volume.

References

1. Abbas JS, Holyoke ED, Moore R, Karakousis CP: The surgical treatment and outcome of soft-tissue sarcoma. Arch Surg 116:765–769, 1981.
2. Akwari OE, Dozois RR, Weiland LH, Beahrs OH: Leiomyosarcoma of the small and large bowel. Cancer 42:1375–1384, 1978.
3. Alvira MM, Mandybur TI, Menefee MG: Light microscopic and ultrastructural observations of a metastasizing malignant epithelioid schwannoma. Cancer 38:1977–1982, 1976.
4. Appleman HD, Helwig EB: Gastric epithelioid leiomyoma and leiomyosarcoma (leiomyoblastoma). Cancer 38:708–728, 1976.
5. Ariel IM, Briceno M: Rhabdomyosarcoma of the extremities and trunk: analysis of 150 patients treated by surgical resection. J Surg Oncol 7:269–287, 1975.
6. Axelson O, Sundell I, Andersson K, Edling C, Hodstedt C, Kling H: Herbicide exposure and tumour mortality. An up-dated epidemiological investigation on Swedish railroad workers. Scand J Work Environ Health 6:73–79, 1980.
7. Beck A: Zur Frage des Röentgensarkoms "Zugleich ein Beitrag zur Pathogenese der Sarkoms." Munchen Med Wschr 69:623–624, 1922.
8. Binder SC, Katz B, Sheridan MFB: Retroperitoneal liposarcoma. Ann Surg 187:257–261, 1978.
9. Cadman CL, Soule EH, Kelly PJ: Synovial sarcoma: an analysis of 134 tumors. Cancer 18:613–627, 1965.
10. Cahan WG, Woodard HQ, Higinbotham NL, Stewart FW, Coley BL: Sarcoma arising in irradiated bone. Report of eleven cases. Cancer 1:3–29, 1948.
11. Cameron HU, Kostuik JP: A long-term follow-up of synovial sarcoma. J Bone Joint Surg 56-B:613–617, 1974.
12. Celik C, Karakousis CP, Moore R, Holyoke ED: Liposarcomas: prognosis and management. J Surg Oncol 14:245–249, 1980.
13. Chen KTK, Kirkegaard DD, Bocian JJ: Angiosarcoma of the breast. Cancer 46:368–371, 1980.

14. Chiotasso PJP, Fazio VW: Prognostic factors of 28 leiomyosarcomas of the small intestine. Surg Gynecol Obstet 155:197–202, 1982.
15. Cody HS, Turnbull AD, Fortner JG, Hajdu SI: The continuing challenge of retroperitoneal sarcomas. Cancer 47:2147–2152, 1981.
16. Coggon D, Acheson ED: Do phenoxy herbicides cause cancer in man? Lancet 1:1057–1059, 1982.
17. Coia LR, Fazekas JT, Kramer S: Postirradiation sarcoma of the head and neck: a report of three late sarcomas following therapeutic irradiation for primary malignancies of the paranasal sinus, nasal cavity, and larynx. Cancer 46:1982–1985, 1980.
18. Cook RR: Dioxin, chloracne, and soft tissue sarcoma. Lancet 1:618–619, 1981.
19. Deck KB, Silberman H: Leiomyosarcomas of the small intestine. Cancer 44:323–325, 1979.
20. DiSant'agnese PA, Knowles DM: Extracardiac rhabdomyoma: a clinicopathologic study and review of the literature. Cancer 46:780–789, 1980.
21. Editorial: Phenoxy herbicides, trichlorophenols, and soft-tissue sarcomas. Lancet 1:1051–1052, 1982.
22. Ekfors TO, Kalino H, Rantakokko V, Latvala M, Parvinen M: Alveolar soft part sarcoma: a report of two cases with some histochemical and ultrastructural observations. Cancer 43:1672–1677, 1979.
23. Enzinger FM, Winslow DJ: Liposarcoma: a study of 103 cases. Virchows Arch Pathol Anat 335:367–388, 1962.
24. Eriksson M, Hardell L, Berg NO, Möller T, Axelson O: Soft tissue sarcomas and exposure to chemical substances: a case-referent study. Br J Indust Med 38:27–33, 1981.
25. Erlandson RA, Woodruff JM: Peripheral nerve sheath tumors: an electron microscopic study of 43 cases. Cancer 49:273–287, 1982.
26. Falk H, Popper H, Thomas LB, Ishak KG: Hepatic angiosarcoma associated with androgenic-anabolic steroids. Lancet 2:1120–1123, 1979.
27. Ferrell HW, Frable WJ: Soft part sarcomas revisited: review and comparison of a second series. Cancer 30:475–480, 1972.
28. Fields JP, Helwig EB: Leiomyosarcoma of the skin and subcutaneous tissue. Cancer 47:156–169, 1981.
29. Gare NF, Lindup R, Strickland P, Bennett MH: Radiation induced fibrosarcoma. Br J Cancer 24:705–711, 1970.
30. Gerner GE, Moore GE: Synovial sarcoma. Ann Surg 181:22–25, 1975.
31. Gerner RE, Moore GE, Pickren JW: Hemangiopericytoma. Ann Surg 179:128–132, 1974.
32. Gerner RE, Moore GE, Pickren JW: Soft tissue sarcomas. Ann Surg 181:803–808, 1975.
33. Ghosh BC, Ghosh L, Huvos AG, Fortner JG: Malignant schwannoma: a clinicopathologic study. Cancer 31:184–190, 1973.
34. Hajdu SI: History and classification of soft tissue tumors. In: Pathology of Soft Tissue Tumors. Philadelphia, Lea & Febiger, 1979, p 44.
35. Hajdu SI, Lemos LB, Kozakewich H, Helson L, Beattie EJ: Growth pattern and differentiation of human soft tissue sarcomas in nude mice. Cancer 47:90–98, 1981.
36. Hajdu SI, Shiu MH, Fortner JG: Tendosynovial sarcoma: a clinicopathological study of 136 cases. Cancer 39:1201–1217, 1977.
37. Hardell L: Soft tissue sarcomas and exposure to phenoxyacetic acids—a clinical observation. Läkartidningen 74:2753–2754, 1977.
38. Hardell L, Sandström A: Case-control study: soft-tissue sarcomas and exposure to phenoxyacetic acids or chlorophenols. Br J Cancer 39:711–717, 1979.
39. Hardy TJ, An T, Brown PW, Terz JJ: Postirradiation sarcoma (malignant fibrous histiocytoma) of axilla. Cancer 42:118–124, 1978.
40. Hare FF, Cerny MJ: Soft tissue sarcoma: a review of 200 cases. Cancer 16:1332–1337, 1963.

41. Hatfield PM, Schulz MD: Postirradiation sarcoma, including 5 cases after x-ray therapy of breast carcinoma. Radiology 96:593–602, 1970.
42. Honchar PA, Halperin WE: 2,4,5-T,trichlorophenol and soft tissue sarcomas. Lancet 1:268–269, 1981.
43. Iwasaki H, Hikuchi M, Takii M, Enjoji M: Benign and malignant fibrous histiocytomas of the soft tissues: functional characterization of the cultured cells. Cancer 50:520–530, 1982.
44. Johnson FE, Kugler MA, Brown SM: Soft tissue sarcomas and chlorinated phenols. Lancet 2:40, 1981.
45. Kearny MM, Soule EH, Ivins JC: Malignant fibrous histiocytoma: a retrospective study of 167 cases. Cancer 45:167–178, 1980.
46. Keyhani A, Booher RJ: Pleomorphic rhabdomyosarcoma. Cancer 5:956–967, 1968.
47. Kinne DW, Chu FCH, Huvos AG, Yagoda A, Fortner JG: Treatment of primary and recurrent retroperitoneal liposarcoma: twenty-five-year experience at Memorial Hospital. Cancer 31:53–64, 1973.
48. Kyriakos M, Kempson RL: Inflammatory fibrous histiocytoma: an aggressive and lethal lesion. Cancer 37:1584–1606, 1976.
49. Leborgne F, Falconi LM: Lymphangiosarcoma of the anterior abdominal wall: a case report. Cancer 46:1228–1230, 1980.
50. Lehti PM, Moseley HS, Peetz ME, Fletcher WS: Liposarcoma of the leg. Am J Surg 144:44–47, 1982.
51. Lieberman PH, Foote FW, Stewart FW, Berg JW: Alveolar soft-part sarcoma. JAMA 198:1047–1051, 1966.
52. Lindsay PC, Ordonez N, Raaf JH: Gastric leiomyosarcoma: clinical and pathological review of fifty patients. J Surg Oncol 18:399–421, 1981.
53. Linscheid RL, Soule EH, Henderson ED: Pleomorphic rhabdomyosarcomata of the extremities and limb girdles: a clinicopathological study. J Bone Joint Surg 47A:715–726, 1965.
54. Maddox JC, Evans HL: Angiosarcoma of skin and soft tissue: a study of forty-four cases. Cancer 48:1907–1921, 1981.
55. Markhede G, Angervall L, Stoner B: A multivariate analysis of the prognosis after surgical treatment of malignant soft-tissue tumors. Cancer 49:1721–1733, 1982.
56. Mathew T: Evidence supporting neural crest origin of an alveolar soft part sarcoma: an ultrastructural study. Cancer 50:507–514, 1982.
57. McMaster MJ, Soule EH, Ivins JC: Hemangiopericytoma: a clinicopathologic study and long-term follow-up of 60 patients. Cancer 36:2232–2244, 1975.
58. McSwain B, Whitehead W, Bennett L: Angiosarcoma: report of three cases of postmastectomy lymphangiosarcoma and one of hemangiosarcoma. South Med J 66:102–106, 1973.
59. Mindell ER, Shah NK, Webster JH: Postradiation sarcoma of bone and soft tissues. Orthop Clin North Am 8:821–834, 1977.
60. Moses M, Selikoff IJ: Soft tissue sarcomas, phenoxy herbicides, and chlorinated phenols. Lancet 1:1370, 1981.
61. Nelson WR, Morfit HM: Lymphangiosarcoma in the lymphedematous arm after radical mastectomy. Cancer 9:1189–1194, 1956.
62. Ott MJ, Holder BB, Olson RD: A mortality analysis of employees engaged in the manufacture of 2,4,5-trichlorophenoxy acetic acid. J Occup Med 22:47–50, 1980.
63. Pack GT, Pierson JC: Liposarcoma. Surgery 36:687–712, 1954.
64. Pack GT, Tabah EJ: Dermatofibrosarcoma protuberans: a report of thirty-nine cases. Arch Surg 62:391–411, 1951.
65. Patchefsky AS, Soriano R, Kostianovsky M: Epithelioid sarcoma: ultrastructural similarity to nodular synovitis. Cancer 39:143–152, 1977.
66. Phillips TL, Sheline GE: Bone sarcomas following radiation therapy. Radiology 81:992–996, 1963.

23

67. Pinkston JA, Sekine I: Postirradiation sarcoma (malignant fibrous histiocytoma) following cervix cancer. Cancer 49:434–438, 1982.

68. Prat J, Woodruff JM, Marcove RC: Epithelioid sarcoma: an analysis of 22 cases indicating the prognostic significance of vascular invasion and regional lymph node metastasis. Cancer 41:1472–1487, 1978.

69. Prioleau PG, Santa Cruz DJ: Lymphangioma circumscriptum following radical mastectomy and radiation therapy. Cancer 42:1989–1991, 1978.

70. Pritchard DJ, Soule EH, Taylor WF, Ivins JC: Fibrosarcoma—a clinicopathologic and statistical study of 199 tumors of the soft tissues of the extremities and trunk. Cancer 33:888–897, 1974.

71. Roth F: Arsen-Leber-Tumoren (Hämangioendotheliom). Z Krebsforsch 61:468–503, 1957.

72. Schrieber H, Barry FM, Russell WC, Macon WL, Ponsky JL, Pories WJ: Stewart-Treves syndrome: a lethal complication of postmastectomy lymphedema and regional immune deficiency. Arch Surg 114:82–85, 1979.

73. Sears HF, Hopson R, Inouye W, Rizzo T, Grotzinger PJ: Analysis of staging and management of patients with sarcoma: a ten-year experience. Ann Surg 191:488–493, 1980.

74. Shieber W, Graham P: An experience with sarcomas of the soft tissues in adults. Surgery 52:295–298, 1962.

75. Shiu MH, Castro EB, Hajdu SI, Fortner JG: Surgical treatment of 297 soft tissue sarcomas of the lower extremity. Ann Surg 182:597–602, 1975.

76. Shiu MH, Farr GH, Papachristou DN, Hajdu SI: Myosarcomas of the stomach: natural history, prognostic factors and management. Cancer 49:177–187, 1982.

77. Shiu MH, McCormack PM, Hajdu, SI, Fortner JG: Surgical treatment of tendosynovial sarcoma. Cancer 43:889–897, 1979.

78. Snover DC, Sumner HW, Dehner LP: Variability of histologic pattern in recurrent soft tissue sarcomas originally diagnosed as liposarcoma. Cancer 49:1005–1015, 1982.

79. Sordillo PP, Chapman R, Hajdu SI, Magill GB, Golbey RB: Lymphangiosarcoma. Cancer 48:1674–1679, 1981.

80. Sordillo PP, Helson L, Hajdu SI, Magill GB, Kosloff C, Golbey RB, Beattie EJ: Malignant schwannoma—clinical characteristics, survival, and response to therapy. Cancer 47:2503–2509, 1981.

81. Soule EH, Geitz M, Henderson ED: Embryonal rhabdomyosarcoma of the limbs and limb girdles: a clinicopathologic study of 61 cases. Cancer 23:1336–1346, 1969.

82. Stewart FW, Treves N: Lymphangiosarcoma in postmastectomy lymphedema: a report of six cases in elephantiasis chirurgica. Cancer 1:64–81, 1948.

83. Storm FK, Eilber FR, Mirra J, Morton DL: Neurofibrosarcoma. Cancer 45:126–129, 1980.

84. Stringel G, Shandling B, Mancer K, Ein EH: Lipoblastoma in infants and children. J Pediatr Surg 17:277–280, 1982.

85. Taxy JB, Battifora H: Malignant fibrous histiocytoma: an electron microscopic study. Cancer 40:254–267, 1977.

86. Thomas LB, Popper H, Berk PD, Selikoff I, Falk H: Vinyl-chloride-induced liver disease: from idiopathic portal hypertension (Banti's syndrome) to angiosarcomas. N Engl J Med 292:17–22, 1975.

87. Travis EL, Kreuther A, Young T, Gerald WL: Unusual postirradiation sarcoma of chest wall. Cancer 38:2269–2273, 1976.

88. Trojanowski JQ, Kleinman GM, Proppe KH: Malignant tumors of nerve sheath origin. Cancer 46:1202–1212, 1980.

89. Underwood JCE, Huck P: Thorotrast associated hepatic angiosarcoma with 36 years latency. Cancer 42:2610–2612, 1978.

90. van Miller JP, Lalich JJ, Allen JR: Increased incidence of neoplasms in rats exposed to low levels of 2,3,7,8-tetrachlorodibenzo-p-dioxin. Chemosphere 6:537–544, 1977.

91. Visfeldt J, Poulson H: On the histopathology of liver and liver tumours in thorium-dioxide patients. Acta Pathol Microbiol Scand (A) 80:97–108, 1972.
92. Weingrad DN, Rosenberg SA: Early lymphatic spread of osteogenic and soft-tissue sarcomas. Surgery 84:231–240, 1978.
93. Weiss SW, Enzinger FM: Malignant fibrous histiocytoma: an analysis of 200 cases. Cancer 41:2250–2266, 1978.
94. Wile AG, Evans HL, Romsdahl MM: Leiomyosarcoma of soft tissue: a clinicopathologic study. Cancer 48:1022–1032, 1981.
95. Yap B-S, Yap H-Y, McBride CM, Bodey GP: Chemotherapy for postmastectomy lymphangiosarcoma. Cancer 47:853–856, 1981.
96. Zack JA, Suskind RS: The mortality experience of workers exposed to tetrachloro-dibenzodioxin in a trichlorophenol process accident. J Occup Med 22:11–14, 1980.

2 Diagnosis and Staging of Soft-Tissue Sarcomas

Optimal management of soft-tissue sarcomas depends upon establishing the diagnosis and determining the extent of both local and systemic disease. The clinical presentation and the procedures employed for these purposes will be reviewed.

Clinical Presentation

Most patients first present with a mass which is usually painless and may have been present for a variable amount of time. Many patients state that the mass first appeared after local trauma and was slowly growing since that time. However, it is most likely that the mass was present prior to the injury; trauma to it merely brought it to the patient's attention. Pain is an unusual symptom of soft-tissue sarcomas; they are usually slow-growing neoplasms and do not have a true capsule with nerve endings which, when stretched, might elicit a sensation of pain. Paresis is a not uncommon symptom and is usually due to involvement of a nerve adjacent to the mass. The patient may complain of swelling distally in the extremity; when present, it is usually due to lymphatic or venous obstruction at a proximal site.

On physical examination the mass should be accurately measured and fixation to bone or adjacent structures determined. This is more easily accomplished when the lesion arises on an extremity, the most frequent primary site for sarcomas in adults. The mass is usually fairly well circumscribed to palpation, although on occasion, especially with retroperitoneal or deep-seated extremity masses, it may be quite diffuse and seem to infiltrate surrounding tissue. Neurovascular involvement can be detected by careful physical examination. Distal pulses, any lymphatic or venous obstruction, and nerve involvement should be carefully sought. Although it is most unusual for soft-tissue sarcomas to metastasize to regional lymph nodes (18), the nodes may be enlarged. Soft, easily movable, well-defined nodes often represent reactive lymphadenitis. Harder, fixed nodes may be due to metastatic sarcoma. Accordingly, a careful nodal examination should be performed on the chance that there has been spread to the regional lymph nodes.

Biopsy Techniques

Treatment planning for the management of soft-tissue sarcomas requires a histologic diagnosis, which must be obtained by biopsy. The sarcoma must also be examined histologically from the standpoint of "grade," since this is a factor affecting proper staging (discussed later). The specific technique of biopsy chosen should be based on the consideration that the mass might be a sarcoma; the surgeon should carefully plan the approach to biopsy so that any subsequent therapeutic operation will not be compromised. The result of not considering a diagnosis of soft-tissue sarcoma might be enucleation of the mass; this approach to a mass of uncertain histology will often compromise the definitive resection of the sarcoma and, therefore, is an approach that should be avoided.

There are four types of biopsy procedures that may be employed to establish the diagnosis of soft-tissue sarcomas: fine needle aspiration, needle biopsy, excisional biopsy, and incisional biopsy.

Fine needle aspirations have been shown to be useful in the diagnosis of many carcinomas, but generally they should not be used for the definitive diagnosis of soft-tissue tumors. Although an aspiration biopsy may demonstrate certain cytologic characteristics consistent with a sarcoma, exact histologic classification may be difficult, and determining the degree of differentiation is essentially impossible. In addition, for well-differentiated tumors, it may not be possible to distinguish a benign from a malignant tumor with confidence. Fine needle aspiration biopsy may, however, be useful in documenting a site of recurrent sarcoma after previous treatment. The treatment plan for primary soft-tissue sarcomas should not be based on aspiration biopsies in most instances.

Needle biopsies are cores of tissue which may be obtained with various types of needle, including Vim-Silverman and Tru-Cut needles. The advantage of obtaining tissue cores is in providing a tissue diagnosis rather than a cytologic diagnosis. By obtaining several cores of tissue, a variety of diagnostic stains can be employed, which may be helpful in histologic characterization of the tumor. In addition, a core can be processed for electron microscopic examination, as these tumors are often difficult to classify by light microscopy.

Excisional biopsy should rarely be performed when a soft-tissue tumor is suspected of being malignant. Excisional biopsy will usually compromise the tissue planes for a subsequent, adequate, soft-part resection. Because the apparent "capsule" surrounding a tumor is, in reality, a pseudocapsule composed of compressed fibrous tissue containing tumor cells, merely enucleating the mass will leave some tumor cells behind and will make it difficult to determine the full extent of tumor and obtain adequate margins at a subsequent operation. Only very small tumors can be excisionally biopsed without altering surrounding tissue planes. The location of the incision itself is also of importance in performing an excisional biopsy (Fig. 2-1). In the extremity the direction of the incision should be along the axis of the involved muscle, and the incision should be limited so that an appropriate ellipse of tissue will include the biopsy wound during a subsequent wider resection.

Incisional biopsy is usually the procedure of choice for obtaining a diagnosis of soft-tissue tumors. The incision should be carefully placed, over the midportion of the tumor, and carried directly down to the tumor so that contamination of adjacent tissue planes is minimized (Fig. 2-2). A large enough specimen of tumor should be obtained to provide for appropriate light and electron microscopic studies. The treatment plan should not be based on a

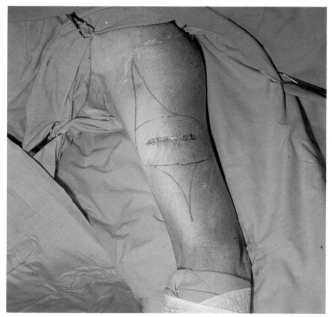

FIG. 2-1.   Patient requiring soft-part resection of a sarcoma of the upper arm. The biopsy incision that was employed to establish the diagnosis was transverse rather than longitudinal, and it complicated both the incision and the design of the skin resection at the time of definitive operation. A longitudinal incision for the biopsy, as demonstrated in Figure 2-2, is preferable for the reasons seen in this photograph.

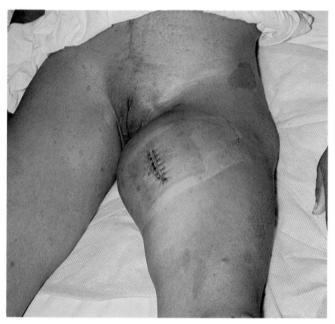

FIG. 2-2.   Patient with malignant fibrous histiocytoma of the proximal thigh demonstrating the limited biopsy incision utilized to establish the diagnosis. The local extent of this sarcoma required hemipelvectomy to achieve adequate soft-tissue margins.

frozen-section report but should await the permanent histologic sections (Fig. 2-3) and, if necessary, the results of electron microscopy. The histologic diagnosis and degree of differentiation should be discussed with the pathologist so appropriate staging (discussed later) and treatment planning can be done.

Imaging Techniques

Optimal management of patients with soft-tissue sarcomas depends upon an accurate delineation of the extent of tumor. After a thorough physical examination and laboratory evaluations, a biopsy is performed and the diagnosis is established. The patient should then undergo various tests to determine whether there is any evidence of metastases and to accurately determine the local extent of the sarcoma.

Posteroanterior and lateral chest radiographs are the most important tests for determining metastatic spread. The first site of sarcoma metastasis is usually pulmonary. About 15% of patients presenting with a primary soft-tissue sarcoma will have pulmonary metastases (17); about two-thirds of these will be detected on routine chest radiographs, and the remainder will be found on whole-lung tomography. The presence of a pulmonary nodule on a chest roentgenogram does not prove the presence of metastatic disease but should be pursued; old radiographs, if available, should be obtained to determine whether the nodule had been previously present. If the nodule is solitary, whole-lung tomography should be performed to determine whether more nodules are present and to search for calcification within the nodule. This may clarify the diagnosis. If the nodule was not present previously and does not have a typical benign appearance, thoracotomy should be performed (prior

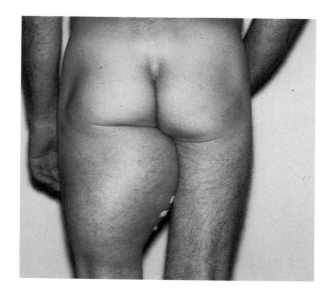

A

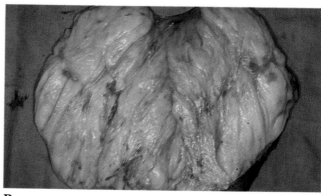

B

FIG. 2-3. Patient with a large soft-tissue mass on the medial posterior thigh (A). The pathologic specimen (B) was a nine-pound benign intramuscular lipoma. This patient clearly demonstrates the value of preliminary biopsy to establish the diagnosis, as the extent of resection in this instance was much more limited and less disabling than it would have been if the actual diagnosis had been sarcoma.

to treatment of the primary tumor) for both diagnosis and treatment (see Chapter 12).

Recently, computed tomography has been evaluated as an adjunct to conventional chest radiography for evaluating the pulmonary parenchyma. Patients evaluated in the Surgery Branch of the National Cancer Institute (4) underwent both whole-lung tomography and computed tomography of the lungs, and the results of these studies were compared with the operative findings. Computed tomography demonstrated 31 nodules not detected on conventional tomography, but only 6 of these represented metastatic sarcoma. Our data confirmed these findings (15), thereby suggesting that computed tomographic scans are more sensitive but less specific than conventional tomography. Thus, when there is a normal chest roentgenogram, abnormal computed tomography should be further evaluated by conventional tomography to determine whether calcification suggestive of a benign granuloma is present. If computed tomography of the chest is normal, there is no need to confirm these findings by whole-lung tomography.

The routine use of radioisotope scans and contrast studies for cancer staging has been evaluated in a series of reports from the National Cancer Institute (1,9,17). Patients with apparently localized cancers who were admitted to the Surgery Branch of the National Cancer Institute during a five and one-half year period underwent liver, bone, brain, and gallium radioisotope scans as well as intravenous pyelography, barium enema, proctosigmoidoscopy, and upper gastrointestinal series. Among patients with sarcomas, these tests did not add to the information gained from history, physical examination, and laboratory evaluation. Thus, it was suggested that these tests should be reserved for those patients with specific clinical indications.

Bitran and co-workers also have investigated the value of gallium scans in a series of patients with sarcomas (3). They found that patients with malignant schwannomas and undifferentiated sarcomas had all known sites of involvement detected by [67]gallium scintigraphy, but patients with other histologic types of sarcoma had many false-negative scans. Although the authors state that these data demonstrate the value of [67]gallium scans, it appears that all

29

sites of metastases were detected by other, more routine diagnostic tests and physical examination, and therefore their data suggest that gallium scans are not particularly useful for the preoperative evaluation of patients with sarcomas.

The value of routine bone scans for determining local bone involvement by soft-tissue sarcomas was investigated in a series of patients by Enneking et al. (8). They reported that ^{99}Tc pyrophosphate or methylene diphosphate was 92% accurate in detecting the presence or absence of contiguous bone involvement by the tumor. However, this was the decisive test in determining the treatment approach in only 1 of 60 patients; most often the scan corroborated other studies. Furthermore, sites of distant metastases were not detected by bone scanning. Thus, although these data purport to demonstrate the value of bone scanning in determining the resectability of soft-tissue sarcomas, the information obtained was usually only confirmatory of the physical examination and other imaging evaluations. Bone scans, therefore, appear to play little role in treatment planning.

Computed tomographic scanning has been recently shown to be effective in both the preoperative assessment and the postoperative follow-up of patients with many types of cancer; it has also been shown to be useful in the evaluation of patients receiving nonoperative therapy. Few studies have investigated its value in the preoperative assessment of the primary tumor in patients with sarcomas by comparing the findings noted on computed tomographic scans with the actual operative findings. An investigation of patients with liposarcoma from the M. D. Anderson Hospital (5) showed that computed tomographic scanning was not useful in providing a histologic diagnosis, but it could be helpful in delineating larger tumor masses than were appreciated by other techniques.

Most other reports have been on the use of computed tomographic scans as a diagnostic modality (19), as compared with other imaging techniques, or as a method to evaluate recurrent tumor. Computed tomographic scans of the primary tumor have been compared with other imaging techniques by several investigators. When computed tomography was compared with ultrasonography (2), the computed tomographic scan was found more accurate than ultrasound, and ultrasound often failed to correctly characterize the internal structure of the mass. In that same study, among 6 patients undergoing arteriography, the arteriogram underestimated the size of the mass in 3 patients. These data were supported by the review of 14 patients from the University of Kansas (13): false negatives were seen with ultrasonography while computed tomographic scans provided more accurate information about relationships of the mass to surrounding structures in the extremity. It was also reported that computed tomographic scans proved more accurate than angiography with the exception of a few distal extremity tumors where there was little surrounding fat. ^{99m}Tc pyrophosphate and ^{67}Ga citrate scans were both found to be significantly less accurate than computed tomographic scans in imaging primary soft-tissue tumors.

We have recently reviewed 46 patients with primary soft-tissue sarcomas to compare the findings on computed tomographic scan with the subsequent findings at operation and in the pathologic specimen (15). The computed tomographic scan appeared most useful for determining the extent of tumor in patients with retroperitoneal primary sites of sarcoma: among 21 patients with primary retroperitoneal tumors, the computed tomographic scan was accurate in 14 of 17 patients undergoing operation and was helpful in the preoperative planning of most of these (Figs. 2-4 and 2-5). There were 3 patients in whom the computed tomography was misleading: 1 patient was

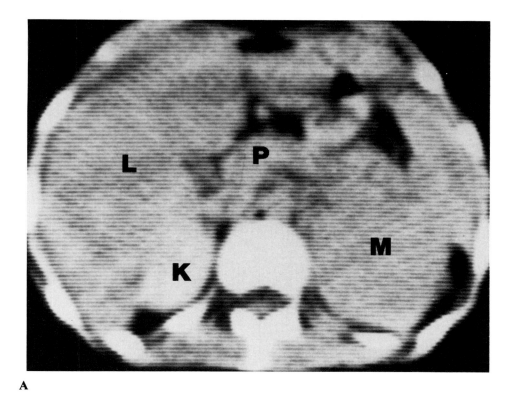

A

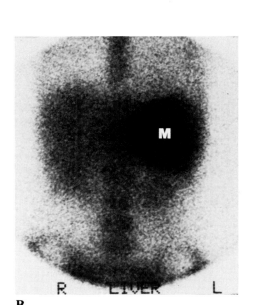

B

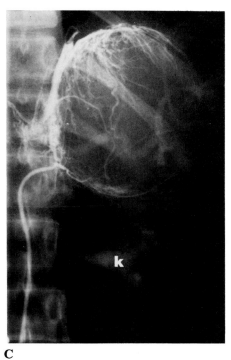

C

FIG. 2-4. **A.** A 15-year-old female presented with nonspecific constitutional symptoms and weight loss. Physical examination was normal. Computed tomography through the liver (*L*), pancreas (*P*), and right kidney (*K*) showed a round left suprarenal mass (*M*); there was no involvement of adjacent structures. **B.** Anteroposterior 48-hour gallium scan showed avid radionuclide uptake in the left upper quadrant mass (*M*). **C.** Selective left middle adrenal artery angiogram showed tumor vessels surrounding the periphery of the tumor superior to the left kidney (*K*). At exploration a left upper quadrant mass, free of all surrounding structures, was excised (Fig. 13-2). Histology was that of a malignant fibrous histiocytoma. Computed tomography had accurately demonstrated lack of involvement of aorta, kidney, and pancreas.

31

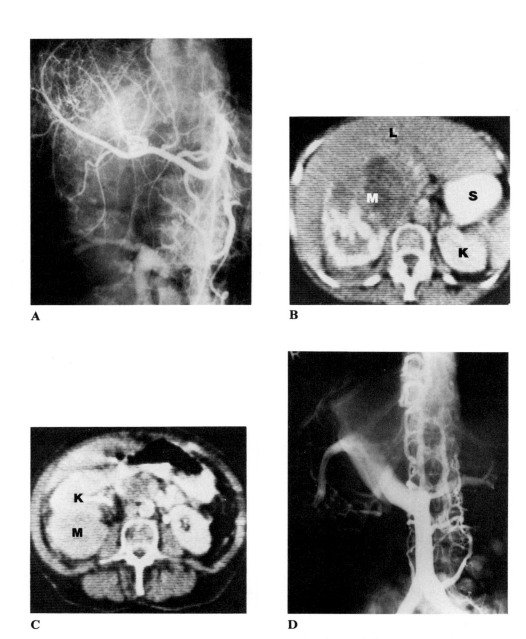

FIG. 2-5. A 67-year-old patient presented with a large right upper quadrant mass thought to be intrahepatic. **A.** Common hepatic artery angiography showed multiple peripheral hepatic artery tumor vessels supplying and draping the mass. **B.** Computed tomographic scan through the liver (*L*), stomach (*S*), and left kidney (*K*) showed a large, partly calcified mass (*M*) which appeared to be intrahepatic at this level. **C.** Computed tomographic scan performed at a lower level showed the retroperitoneal origin of the mass (*M*), demonstrated by the anterior displacement of the right kidney (*K*). **D.** Inferior vena cavagram showed marked right lateral displacement and interruption of the vena cava with multiple collateral veins bypassing the obstruction.

The demonstration of the retroperitoneal nature of the mass by computed tomography suggested that the vena cava was involved by tumor, thus resulting in the vena cavagram. This preoperative evaluation allowed positioning of the patient to resect the vena cava with the mass and replace the vena cava with a graft. The patient remains free of recurrence three years later.

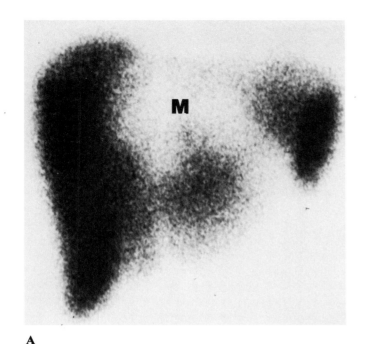

A

FIG. 2-6. This 19-year-old female had a history of taking oral contraceptives. She presented with a large epigastric mass. **A.** Anteroposterior view of the liver-spleen scan showed a photon-deficient mass in the left lobe of the liver. **B.** Transverse ultrasound through the liver (*L*) and kidneys (*K*) showed a large mixed echogenic solid mass (*arrows*) anterior to the inferior vena cava (*C*). **C.** Computed tomographic scan through the liver (*L*), kidneys (*K*), and stomach (*S*) showed a hypodense mass (*M*) which appeared to be intrahepatic.

At exploration a leiomyosarcoma arising from the stomach was found; the left lobe of the liver was displaced anteriorly but was not involved by tumor.

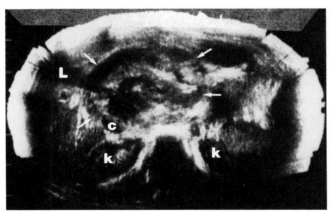

B

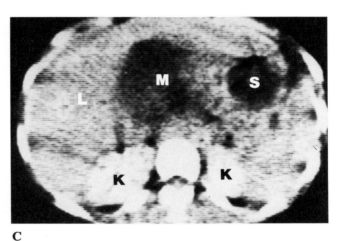

C

thought to have a liver tumor (Fig. 2-6) but at operation was found to have a leiomyosarcoma of the stomach with adherence to the liver. Two patients had more extensive sarcoma at operation than was demonstrated on computed tomographic scan: 1 had a leiomyosarcoma extending from the left side of the retroperitoneum into the porta hepatis, and the other had a mesenteric mass that was not demonstrated on the computed tomographic scan.

Computed tomographic scans were especially useful in following patients after resection of retroperitoneal sarcomas. Among 12 patients with follow-up CT scans, 6 had recurrence of the tumor first detected by the computed tomographic scan. Two patients had a response to chemotherapy that was documented by the computed tomographic scan, and 3 patients had normal computed tomography and no clinical evidence of recurrence. One patient had a false-positive computed tomographic scan: six months after resection of a left upper abdominal malignant fibrous histiocytoma (accurately detected and delineated by computed tomography), a routine computed tomographic scan demonstrated a mass in the region of the previous tumor bed. Exploration demonstrated only scar tissue. These data suggest that computed tomographic scans are useful for the follow-up evaluation of patients with retroperitoneal

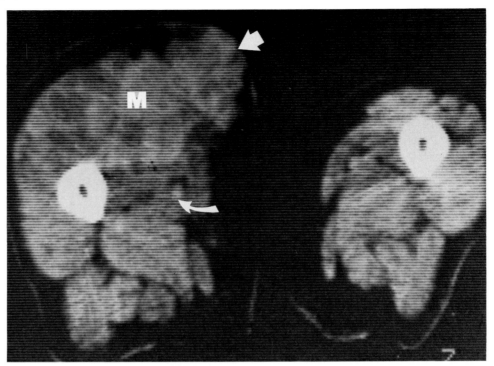

FIG. 2-7.   A 61-year-old woman presented with an 18 cm anterior thigh mass several months after enucleation of a liposarcoma. Computed tomographic scan through both thighs showed an anterior compartment mass (*M*) with extension into the subcutaneous fat (*arrowhead*); the mass appeared to surround the contrast-filled femoral vessels (*curved arrow*). Clinical examination suggested the tumor was mobile; the vessels were explored and found to be free of tumor (Fig. 5-11B), with a normal tissue plane present. Resection of the quadriceps could be performed, thus preserving a functional leg.

sarcomas, but a baseline computed tomographic scan should be obtained in the early postoperative period to prevent later problems in interpretation.

Among 16 patients with extremity soft-tissue sarcomas, computed tomography was accurate for determination of extent of tumor in 10 but only helpful (beyond what was found on clinical examination) in 2. In these patients with proximal arm sarcomas, computed tomography demonstrated chest wall involvement which was not clinically apparent. In 2 patients it overestimated the extent of the tumor; both patients would have undergone hemipelvectomy if exploration had not been undertaken because of the clinical findings suggesting feasibility of soft part resection (Fig. 2-7). Overestimation of tumor size with the suggestion of neurovascular involvement in these cases appeared to be due to edema of muscle surrounding the tumor (6,7,12). Four other patients did not undergo resection, owing to the presence of metastatic sarcoma, but computed tomographic scans correlated well with the clinical findings. Therefore, computed tomographic scans appeared to be useful in proximal extremity tumors but were not useful in the evaluation of other extremity sites (10) and were, at times, misleading.

Postoperative computed tomographic scans of the operative field in the extremity were performed in four patients (Fig. 2-8); one detected an iliac node metastasis in a patient following a soft-part resection of a lateral thigh fibrosarcoma. In other patients the computed tomographic scans of the primary site in the extremity following resection were of no clinical value.

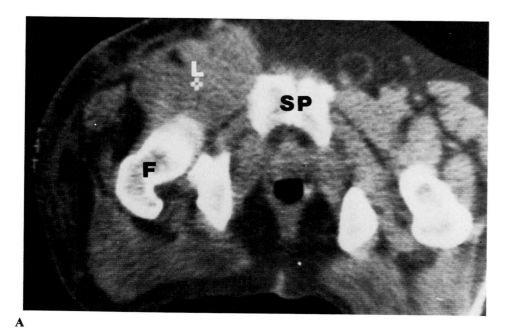

A

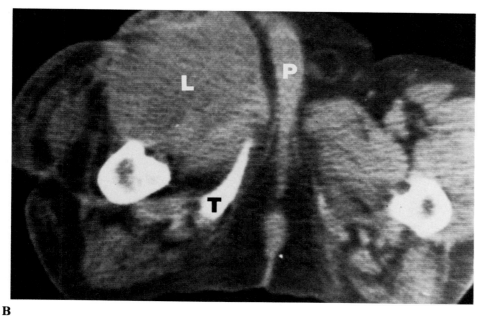

B

FIG. 2-8. A 60-year-old male had previously undergone soft-part resection and radiation therapy for a liposarcoma of the upper thigh (Fig. 11-1). He presented with a large upper thigh mass which was difficult to evaluate on clinical grounds owing to the scarring and previous radiation therapy. **A.** Computed tomography performed through the symphysis pubis (*SP*) and femoral neck (*F*) showed recurrent liposarcoma (*L*) in the right inguinal area. **B.** At the level of the ischial tuberosity (*T*) the liposarcoma (*L*) appeared separate from the base of the penis. The patient underwent a hemipelvectomy, using the computed tomographic scan as guidelines, and had negative margins on the specimen.

Computed tomographic scans of primary trunk or abdominal wall tumors were very useful in delineating tumor extent. Among four patients undergoing resection, scans demonstrated more advanced tumors and deeper extension, such as rib involvement, than could be detected upon physical examination. Computed tomographic scans were also useful in detecting recurrence following resection, despite normal clinical examination and routine radiographs.

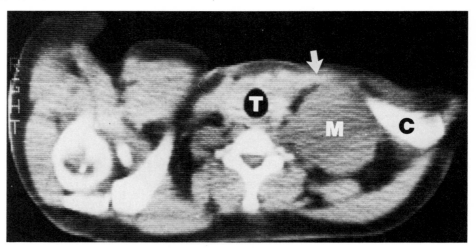

A

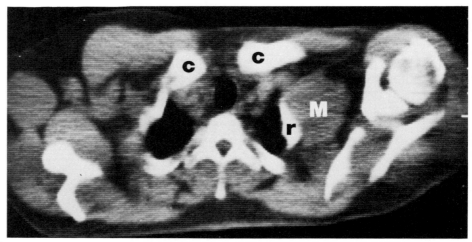

B

FIG. 2-9. A 39-year-old patient with neurofibromatosis presented with a left supra-clavicular mass that was biopsied as a neurofibrosarcoma. **A.** Computed tomography through the thyroid gland, trachea (*T*), and left clavicle (*C*) showed a large mass (*M*) in the supraclavicular fossa elevating the sternocleidomastoid muscle (*arrow*). **B.** At the level of the medial clavicular heads (*C*), superior mediastinum, lung apices, and first rib (*R*) the scan showed the mass (*M*) abutting the chest wall. At exploration the sarcoma was found to arise from the brachial plexus and was free of the chest wall and spine. An interscapulothoracic amputation was performed.

Patients with primary head and neck soft-tissue sarcomas have limited fatty tissue for delineation of tissue planes and the neoplastic mass (Fig. 2-9). Among four patients, computed tomographic scans underestimated tumor size in two. Thus, if the physical findings contradict the computed tomographic scan, we feel that exploration should be undertaken to determine tumor extent prior to major ablative surgery. Computed tomography is, however, particularly useful in the evaluation of sarcomas located above the mandible, an area difficult to evaluate by either physical examination or conventional radiography.

The histology of soft-tissue sarcomas could not be predicted by computed tomography. Although leiomyosarcomas tended to have multiple areas of decreased density, due to hemorrhage and tumor necrosis, this appearance was not diagnostic. In addition, computed tomographic scans did not appear to be more or less useful for any individual histologic type of sarcoma. Com-

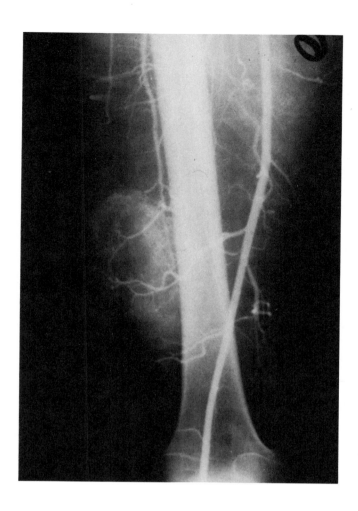

FIG. 2-10. Arteriogram of a patient with liposarcoma arising in the distal quadriceps muscle. It is obvious from this study that the superficial femoral artery is clear of this lesion, which was subsequently treated by soft-tissue resection of the quadriceps muscle group.

puted tomography did, however, appear useful in evaluating lipomas arising within muscles of an extremity, masses difficult to evaluate by physical examination which could be easily mistaken for malignant tumors. Eight such patients underwent computed tomographic scan with the demonstration of the typical consistency of normal fat; the six masses subsequently excised were proven to be lipomas. Nevertheless, because two well-differentiated retroperitoneal liposarcomas had the same density as fat on computed tomography, a biopsy should be performed in such instances to confirm the histologic type of the tumor.

Angiography has been a popular method of evaluating soft-tissue sarcomas prior to surgery, but may now be passing out of favor owing to its limited accuracy when compared with computed tomography. Prior to the availability of computed tomographic scans, angiography was frequently used at our institution (Fig. 2-10). Hudson et al. (11) studied 56 patients with extremity soft-tissue sarcomas and found the angiogram helpful in only 36; there was no correlation with the histology of the tumor. In addition, there is no mention of how many patients had helpful information demonstrated by angiography above what was demonstrated clinically; this study was performed before the computed tomography era. Six patients had arteriograms that were frankly misleading and underestimated the extent of tumor.

Ekelund et al. (7) studied 21 patients with soft-tissue sarcomas arising in an extremity. They found that angiography correctly evaluated tumor size in 17 of 21 patients and computed tomography in 15 of 21 patients; however, considering only factors important for surgical planning, angiography was useful in 8 patients and computed tomography in 14 patients. They favored computed tomography as the initial imaging test. Among 4 patients in our recent series who had arteriography as well as computed tomographic scan, the arteriogram demonstrated tumor in all patients but in no patient did it demonstrate the relationships to normal structures demonstrated by computed tomography (Figs. 2-4 and 2-5). Thus, the role of angiography appears limited in patients with extremity soft-tissue sarcomas.

Lowman et al. (14) investigated the angiographic patterns of primary retroperitoneal tumors and showed that many derived their blood supply from the lumbar arteries. This information could be useful to determine whether a tumor is retroperitoneal but we have not found it useful in planning the operative resection of these tumors. The use of computed tomographic scans has relegated the angiogram to a minor role in delineating the extent of retroperitoneal soft-tissue sarcomas.

Staging

A major problem in the evaluation of reported results of treatment of soft-tissue sarcomas has been the heterogeneity of the patient populations studied. Accurate staging is necessary for protocol development, to provide quality control of data, and to report end results. The American Joint Committee for Cancer Staging and End Results Reporting reported 1215 patients with soft-tissue sarcomas studied at 13 institutions to develop a useful staging system for these tumors (19).

The initial goal of this study was to prepare a staging system based on the TNM system (primary tumor, regional lymph nodes, distant metastases). However, it soon became apparent that the biologic behavior of sarcomas depended heavily on the degree of differentiation of the tumor; accordingly, tumor grade (G) was added, thus providing for a TNMG system. The schema for staging soft-tissue sarcomas is shown in Table 2-1, and the stage grouping for soft-tissue sarcomas is shown in Table 2-2.

When all patients with soft-tissue sarcomas had their survival calculated according to stage, a good correlation was observed (Table 2-3). Similarly, when the histologic types were subclassified according to stage, prognosis decreased with increasing stage. It should be noted that, although histologic grading is an important part of staging, it is not necessary for stage III or stage IV. In addition, it was found that most rhabdomyosarcomas, angiosarcomas, and synovial sarcomas were high-grade and therefore at least stage III even if no metastases had occurred; thus, the prognosis was poor with these tumor types no matter what the clinical stage of the tumor. Patients with

Table 2-1.   Schema for Staging Soft-Tissue Sarcomas by TNMG (16)

T	Primary tumor
	T_1 Tumor less than 5 cm
	T_2 Tumor 5 cm or greater
	T_3 Tumor that grossly invades bone, major vessel, or major nerve
N	Regional lumph nodes
	N_0 No histologically verified metastasis to regional lymph nodes
	N_1 Histologically verified regional lymph node metastasis
M	Distant metastasis
	M_0 No distant metastasis
	M_1 Distant metastasis
G	Histologic grade of malignancy
	G_1 Low
	G_2 Moderate
	G_3 High

Table 2-2. Stage Grouping for Soft-Tissue Sarcomas (16)

Stage I

Stage Ia

$G_1T_1N_0M_0$ Grade 1 tumor less than 5 cm in diameter with no regional lymph node or distant metastases

Stage Ib

$G_1T_2N_0M_0$ Grade 1 tumor 5 cm or greater in diameter with no regional lymph node or distant metastases

Stage II

Stage IIa

$G_2T_1N_0M_0$ Grade 2 tumor less than 5 cm in diameter with no regional lymph node or distant metastases

Stage IIb

$G_2T_2N_0M_0$ Grade 2 tumor 5 cm or greater in diameter with no regional lymph node or distant metastases

Stage III

Stage IIIa

$G_3T_1N_0M_0$ Grade 3 tumor less than 5 cm in diameter with no regional lymph node or distant metastases

Stage IIIb

$G_3T_2N_0M_0$ Grade 3 tumor 5 cm or greater in diameter with no regional lymph node or distant metastases

Stage IIIc

Any $GT_{1-2}N_1M_0$ Tumor of any grade or size (no invasion) with regional lymph node but no distant metastases

Stage IV

Stage IVa

Any $GT_3N_{0-1}M_0$ Tumor of any grade that grossly invades bone, major vessel, or major nerve with or without regional lymph node metastases but without distant metastases

Stage IVb

Any $GTNM_1$ Tumor with distant metastases

---

unclassified tumors, which by inference were high-grade, also did poorly. Thus, in general, with the exceptions just noted, this staging system appears to be reasonably accurate in predicting prognosis in patients with soft-tissue sarcomas.

Table 2-3. Soft-Tissue Sarcoma, Survival by Stage (16)

	No. of cases	Percent surviving*			
		1 year	2 years	5 years	10 years
All stages	1215	74%	58%	41%	30%
Complete staging information	702	73	55	40	30
Stage I	177	91	84	75	63
IA	55	98	93	(83)	(75)
IB	122	88	80	72	(58)
Stage II	86	87	74	(55)	(40)
IIA	29	(90)	(79)	(59)	(41)
IIB	57	86	(72)	(53)	(40)
Stage III	329	71	47	29	19
IIIA	69	84	(61)	42	27
IIIB	211	68	46	26	16
IIIC	49	(65)	(34)	(23)	(23)
Stage IV	110	37	19	7	3

* ( ) = standard errors between 5% and 10%.

39

References

1. Bagley DH, Felix EL, Sindelar WF, Doppman JL, Ketcham AS: Barium enema, proctosigmoidoscopy, and upper gastrointestinal series in the preoperative evaluation of the cancer patient. Cancer 39:1743–1747, 1977.

2. Bernardino ME, Jing B-S, Thomas JL, Lindell MM, Zornoza J: The extremity soft-tissue lesion: a comparative study of ultrasound, computed tomography, and xeroradiography. Radiology 139:53–59, 1981.

3. Bitran JD, Bekerman C, Golomb HM, Simon MA: Scintigraphic evaluation of sarcomata in children and adults by Ga^{67} citrate. Cancer 42:1760–1765, 1978.

4. Chang AE, Schaner EG, Conkle DM, Flye MW, Doppman JL, Rosenberg SA: Evaluation of computed tomography in the detection of pulmonary metastases: a prospective study. Cancer 43:913–916, 1979.

5. deSantos LA, Ginaldi S, Wallace S: Computed tomography in liposarcoma. Cancer 47:46–54, 1981.

6. Eglund N, Ekelund F, Sako M, Persson B: CT of soft tissue tumors. Am J Roentgenol 137:725–729, 1981.

7. Ekelund L, Herrlin K, Rydholm A: Comparison of computed tomography and angiography in the evaluation of soft tissue tumors of the extremities. Acta Radiol Diagn 23:15–28, 1982.

8. Enneking WF, Chew FS, Springfield DS, Hudson TM, Spanier SS: The role of radionuclide bone-scanning in determining the resectability of soft-tissue sarcomas. J Bone Joint Surg 63-A:249–257, 1981.

9. Felix EL, Bagley DH, Sindelar WF, Johnston GS, Ketcham AS: The value of the liver scan in preoperative screening of patients with malignancies. Cancer 38:1137–1141, 1976.

10. Heelan RT, Watson RC, Smith J: Computed tomography of lower extremity tumors. Am J Roentgenol 132:933–937, 1979.

11. Hudson TM, Haas G, Enneking WF, Hawkins JF: Angiography in the management of musculoskeletal tumors. Surg Gynecol Obstet 141:11–21, 1975.

12. Jones ET, Kuhns LR: Pitfalls in the use of computed tomography for musculoskeletal tumors in children. J Bone Joint Surg 63-A:1297–1304, 1981.

13. Levine E, Lee KR, Neff JR, Maklad NF, Robinson RG, Preston DF: Comparison of computed tomography and other imaging modalities in the evaluation of musculoskeletal tumors. Radiology 131:431–437, 1979.

14. Lowman RM, Grnja V, Peck DR, Osborn D, Love L: The angiographic patterns of the primary retroperitoneal tumors: the role of the lumbar arteries. Radiology 104:259–268, 1972.

15. Neifeld JP, Walsh JW, Lawrence W: Computed tomography in the management of soft tissue tumors. Surg Gynecol Obstet 155:535–540, 1982.

16. Russell WO, Cohen J, Enzinger F, Hajdu SI, Heise H, Martin RG, Meissner W, Miller WT, Schmitz RL, Suit HD: A clinical and pathological staging system for soft tissue sarcomas. Cancer 40:1562–1570, 1977.

17. Sindelar WF, Bagley DH, Felix EL, Doppman JL, Ketcham AS: Lung tomography in cancer patients: full-lung tomograms in screening for pulmonary metastases. JAMA 240:2060–2063, 1978.

18. Weingrad DN, Rosenberg SA: Early lymphatic spread of osteogenic and soft-tissue sarcomas. Surgery 84:231–240, 1978.

19. Wilson JS, Korobkin M, Genant HK, Bovill EG: Computed tomography of musculoskeletal disorders. Am J Roentgenol 131:55–61, 1978.

Surgical Treatment of Soft-Tissue Sarcomas in Adults

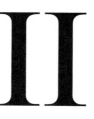

Operative Treatment of Soft-Part Sarcomas

3

Although soft-part sarcomas are radiosensitive, their rate of curability by radiation alone is limited, and surgical resection is accepted as the treatment of choice for most primary tumors. Adjuvant therapy with radiation might well affect the scope of the operation employed, and the data available for defining the value of this adjuvant treatment will be discussed in Chapter 11. The major treatment decision for sarcomas relates to the extent of surgical resection employed, a factor primarily dictated by the anatomic relationships of the individual tumor. Most sarcomas arise in an extremity where a decision regarding amputation must be made. The key principle of resection is that of achieving surgical margins adequate to prevent local treatment failure. In this regard there is some degree of uncertainty as to how wide the gross margins must be, whether total compartmental excision is always required, and the possible role of the histologic grade of the sarcoma in the choice of operative procedure. The heterogeneity of sarcomas, from the standpoint of histologic types, histologic grades, and anatomic locations, does make definition of the optimal operation difficult, but the procedures illustrated in subsequent chapters will serve as general guides for the surgeon.

Many soft-part neoplasms have the misleading appearance of being encapsulated. This "pseudoencapsulation" is usually described by the pathologist as a compressed rim of fibrous tissue containing sarcoma cells at the periphery of the ever-expanding tumor. This gross pathologic feature suggesting a capsule could lead the inexperienced surgeon to enucleate the tumor without achieving a clear margin of normal tissue. Because this rim of fibrous tissue will almost surely contain sarcoma cells, such a procedure, when performed instead of a preliminary biopsy, leads to a high incidence of local recurrence if this is the only resection employed (2). Also, this initial approach seriously jeopardizes the chance of permanent local control of the neoplasm by a subsequent, more adequate procedure, owing to the frequent inability to be certain of resecting the entire potentially involved area at the time of secondary resection. Proper operative management requires resection of the neoplastic mass with an adequate envelope of normal tissue to decrease the chance of local recurrence (1,4,8). This resection will include skin, subcutaneous tissue, adjacent muscle and fibrous tissue, and the biopsy site itself. To adhere to this principle in the extremities, it is often both appropriate and necessary to remove the major portion of a muscle group or muscle compartment. Some consider

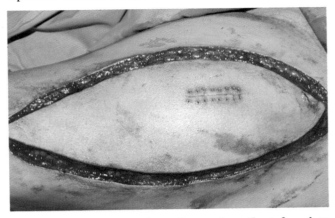

FIG. 3-1. Operative view of a male patient found to have a soft-tissue sarcoma arising in the musculature of the lateral thigh distal to the anterior iliac spine. The scar in the center of the tissue to be resected is from the biopsy incision employed for diagnosis.

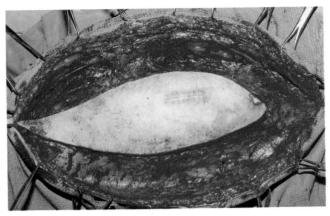

FIG. 3-2. Skin flaps have been dissected to allow resection of a generous margin of muscle around the sarcoma. Wide gross tissue margins producing a generous muscle "envelope" around the sarcoma lead essentially to total resection of the muscle compartment involved. Resection is carried out from the origins to the insertions of the relevant muscles.

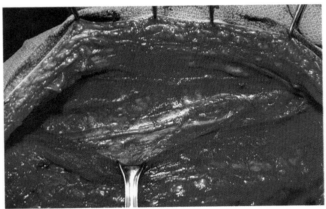

FIG. 3-3. The anterior plane of dissection in this instance is along the femoral vessels. These are found to be well away from the primary site of the sarcoma, and there is a large margin of muscle tissue between these vessels and the lesion.

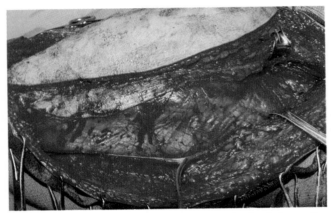

FIG. 3-4. The fascia lata has been incised laterally, thereby exposing the vastus lateralis muscle, which contains the actual sarcoma.

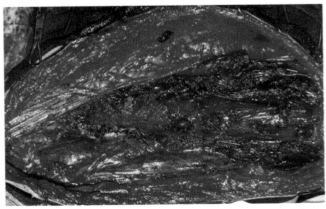

FIG. 3-5. Resection of the large muscle mass has been completed without exposing the sarcoma at any point during the dissection. This view demonstrates the femur in the depth of the operative defect and the femoral vessels at the anterior margin of the dissection.

44

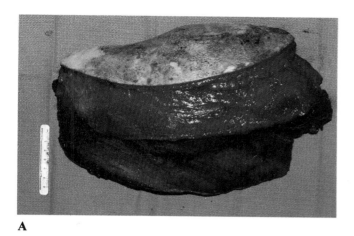

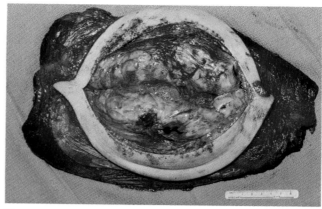

A   **B**

FIG. 3-6. The operative specimen (**A**) and the sarcoma with a muscle envelope as seen when the overlying skin is bisected (**B**).

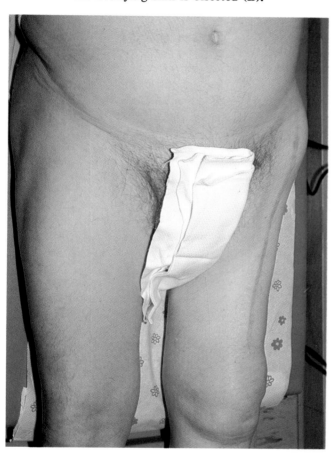

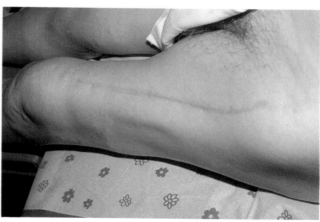

B

FIG. 3-7. The healed wound after rehabilitation of the patient. The soft-tissue defect is apparent when compared with the contralateral thigh (**A**). The femur is palpable just below the scar of the skin closure seen in **B**.

A

this radical compartmental resection much more capable of ensuring local control than a more simple wide en bloc resection with gross tissue margins (4), particularly with high-grade lesions. Superiority of total compartmental resection over a wide resection, when a sarcoma arises within such a compartment, is difficult to establish. However, a practical point is that the proximal and distal portions of a muscle group that is widely resected centrally have no useful function after postoperative recovery. For this reason soft-part resections with truly adequate gross margins are either total compartmental resections or very similar in scope. An example of this approach to soft-tissue resection for sarcomas is illustrated in Figures 3-1 to 3-7.

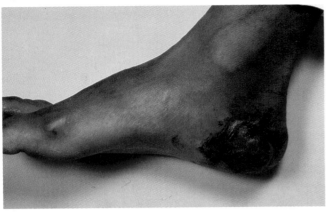

FIG. 3-8. Unusual soft-tissue sarcoma (clear cell sarcoma) arising from aponeurosis of calcaneal region in a 25-year-old male.

Sarcomas close to the joints or bones or adherent to major neurovascular structures, particularly in the distal portion of an extremity, or tumors overlying the shoulder or pelvic girdle, often must be removed by amputation to achieve adequate margins. There are some exceptions to this, such as the anatomic area over the wing of the scapula or the buttock, and an attempt to achieve a radical resection of the sarcoma in these sites is obviously prefera-

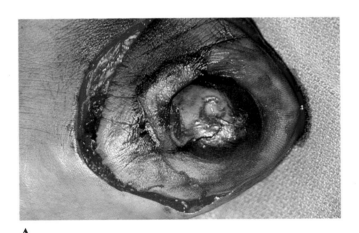

A

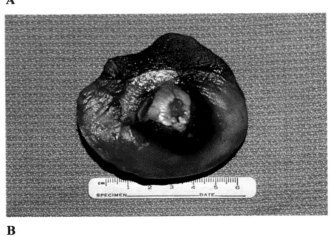

B

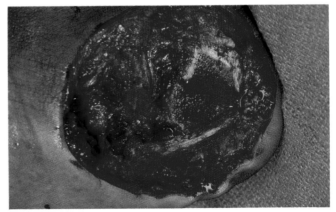

C

FIG. 3-9. Wide local resection including portion of calcaneus underlying the lesion was selected in lieu of amputation (**A**). The surgical specimen (**B**) demonstrated free margins on pathologic study. The operative defect after resection shows the transected surface of the calcaneus in the base of the wound (**C**). Wound closure was accomplished with a split-thickness graft, and the patient has remained well three years postoperative.

ble to amputation if adequate margins can be achieved. There are occasional atypical presentations that may be suitable for nonamputative surgical resections (Fig. 3-8 to 3-9). Despite the major interest that all of us have in "limb salvage," compromise in the attempt to achieve clear margins, just to preserve the limb (or its vascular supply), will usually result in failure of local tumor control. The incidence of local treatment failure in patients with microscopically involved margins is high even if adjuvant radiotherapy is employed (7,9), although less than optimal gross margins may prove satisfactory in some patients who receive postoperative radiation as part of the treatment plan (6,7,10) (see Chapter 11). These concerns regarding extent of operation and the question of preoperative or postoperative irradiation only relate to the adequacy of local control; but local treatment failure is best avoided, as it may allow distant metastasis before the local failure is clinically evident (2,8).

Some surgeons are reluctant to consider radical or wide soft-part resection in lieu of an amputation for most sarcomas on the extremities because of the old and incorrect concept that a large number of these sarcomas are multicentric in origin. It is our view that the primary consideration in the surgical treatment must be complete confidence regarding the adequacy of surgical margins. Wide soft-part resection can achieve this in most instances, but there was a 17% local recurrence rate with wide resection for previously untreated patients in the series of lower extremity sarcomas reported from Memorial Hospital (8), while a lower local failure rate occurred with amputation (7%). The histogenetic classification or histologic grade may temper the decision regarding the choice of amputation versus a nonamputative operative procedure, but this is usually a secondary consideration, despite the higher local failure rate that is observed after operation for high-grade lesions. The principle of including an adequate envelope of normal tissue around the sarcoma applies to less common primary sites, such as the head and neck, trunk, or retroperitoneum, but the option of resection by amputation is obviously not available.

The regional lymph nodes may be a site of metastasis of soft-tissue sarcomas, but the frequency is low for most histologic types in adults (see Chapter 13 regarding special features of childhood sarcomas). Elective lymph node dissection does not seem indicated in the management of most soft-part sarcomas, since the incidence of nodal metastases is much too low to justify the morbidity of the procedure unless there is clinical lymphadenopathy or the primary lesion is anatomically situated over a lymph node basin. Practically speaking, nonpalpable regional lymph nodes are included in the dissection, or with an amputation, only if these can be removed without additional risk or disability. On the basis of the reported frequency of metastases to regional lymph nodes summarized from past series (5,10), it may be an advantage to dissect regional lymph nodes in patients with high-grade synovial sarcomas or malignant fibrous histiocytomas, but no valid clinical trials have established this approach as beneficial.

The specific operations for sarcomas in various anatomic sites depicted in the following chapters are based on the general principles just discussed. All operations described are based on the concept of wide soft-part resection, with resection of generous margins of normal tissue around the gross neoplasm, but these operations are frequently very similar to total compartmental resection for many anatomic sites for the reasons discussed. Standard amputations sometimes required to achieve adequate surgical margins are not depicted, as these are familiar to most surgeons, but the less commonly employed major amputations are described.

47

References

1. Bowden L, Booher RJ: The principles and technique of resection of soft parts for sarcoma. Surgery 44:963–977, 1958.
2. Cantin J, McNeer GP, Chu F, Booher RJ: The problem of local recurrence after treatment of soft tissue sarcoma. Ann Surg 168:47–53, 1968.
3. Devereux DF, Wilson RE, Corson JM, Antman KH, Greenberger JS: Surgical treatment of low grade soft tissue sarcomas. Am J Surg 143:490–494, 1982.
4. Enneking WF, Spanier SS, Malawer MM: The effect of the anatomic setting on the results of surgical procedures for soft parts sarcoma of the thigh. Cancer 47:1005–1022, 1981.
5. Lee Y-TN, Moore TN, Schwinn CP: Metastasis of sarcomatous lesion in regional lymph node. J Surg Oncol 20:53–58, 1982.
6. Lindberg RD, Martin RG, Romsdahl MM, Barkley HT: Conservative surgery and postoperative radiotherapy in 300 adults with soft tissue sarcomas. Cancer 47:2391–2397, 1981.
7. Rosenberg SA: Treatment of soft tissue sarcomas. *In* Lawrence W Jr, Ghosh B (eds): Surgical Oncology Research Workshop. NIH Publication No. 82–2444, September 9, 1981.
8. Shiu MH, Castro ElB, Hajdu SI, Fortner JG: Surgical treatment of 297 soft tissue sarcomas of the lower extremities. Ann Surg 182:597–602, 1975.
9. Suit HD, Proppe KH, Mankin HJ, Wood WC: Preoperative radiation therapy for sarcoma of soft tissue. Cancer 47:2269–2274, 1981.
10. Weingrad DN, Rosenberg SA: Early lymphatic spread of osteogenic and soft tissue sarcomas. Surgery 84:231–240, 1978.

Operations for Sarcomas on the Upper Extremity

4

The general principles of soft-part resection apply to sarcomas arising in the upper extremity, but the relative proportion of patients requiring amputation is greater than with sarcomas in the lower extremities. The smaller muscle masses in the arm and forearm, when compared with the thigh and leg, do not allow as wide a soft-tissue margin around the sarcoma and, in many instances, this prevents limb preservation. Nevertheless, the soft-tissue resections for arm and forearm sites are described and illustrated. In each instance the procedure essentially includes resection of the entire muscle compartment and fits the category of radical compartmental resection, since this is usually required to achieve an adequate gross margin. When amputation is required, the standard techniques are employed for midarm and distal sites, but interscapulothoracic amputation is indicated for more proximal sites.

Soft-Part Resection for Sarcoma of the Forearm

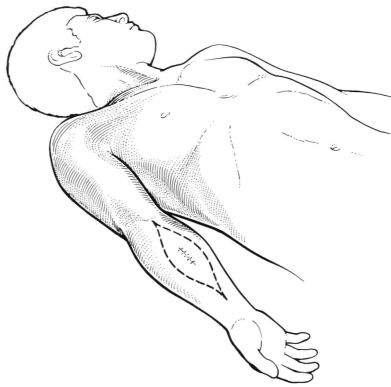

FIG. 4-1. The patient is in the supine position with arm, forearm, and hand in a sterile field. The skin incision around the biopsy wound is outlined.

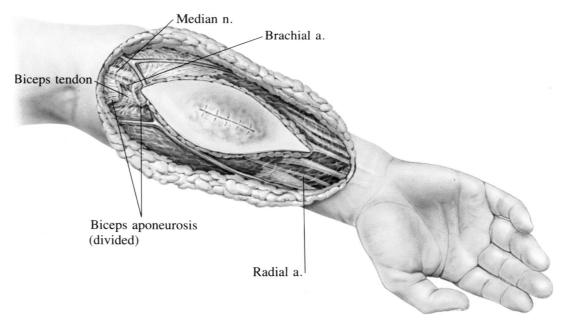

FIG. 4-2. A vertical elliptical incision is made from the antecubital fossa to the lower third of the forearm, circumventing the skin and subcutaneous tissues in the region of the biopsy site. The actual dissection will depend on the specific anatomic site of the sarcoma; the procedure for a volar lesion will be described. Skin flaps are developed at the level of the fascia, and the bicipital aponeurosis is divided.

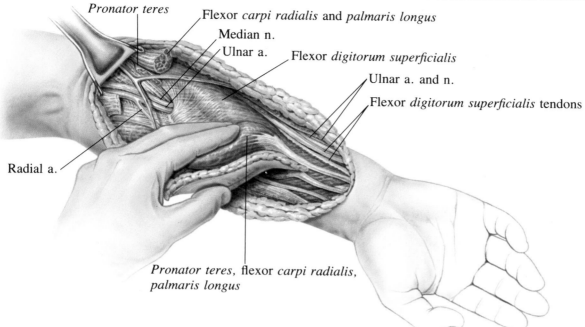

Pronator teres

Flexor *carpi radialis* and *palmaris longus*

Median n.

Ulnar a.

Flexor *digitorum superficialis*

Ulnar a. and n.

Flexor *digitorum superficialis* tendons

Radial a.

Pronator teres, flexor *carpi radialis*, palmaris longus

FIG. 4-3.   After dividing the bicipital aponeurosis, the median nerve and the brachial artery are identified. The pronator teres, flexor carpi radialis, and the palmaris longus are divided at their origins, exposing the flexor digitorum superficialis. This muscle will be detached from its origin as the next step in the dissection.

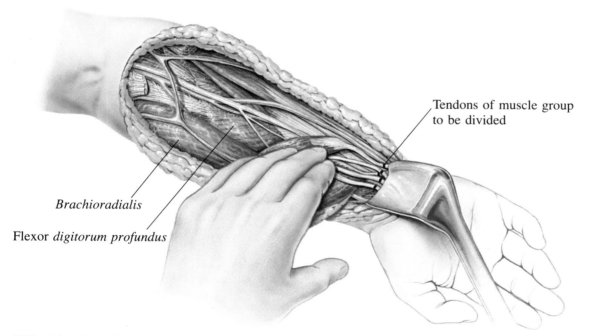

Tendons of muscle group to be divided

Brachioradialis

Flexor *digitorum profundus*

FIG. 4-4.   Detachment of the origin of the flexor digitorum superficialis will expose the ulnar nerve and artery, as well as the radial artery and median nerve. If the tumor mass is well contained in this compartment, the dissection of this muscle group is carried distally toward the wrist, and the specimen is removed en bloc after dividing the distal tendons at the level of the wrist. However, if the tumor mass extends beyond the anterior compartment to the flexor digitorum profundus, most likely the ulnar nerve and artery should be sacrificed. Diffuse extension of the tumor to involve the interosseous membrane is a definite indication for amputation.

51

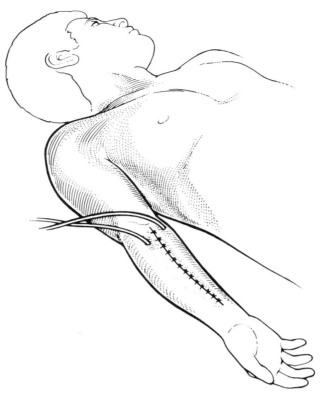

FIG. 4-5. The wound is closed in two layers with interrupted sutures. Suction drainage and a cock-up plaster splint are useful for early postoperative management. Rehabilitation depends, in part, upon the structures sacrificed but a functional hand remains. If the ulnar nerve is sacrificed, a sensory deficit will be present, but this is usually not a major problem.

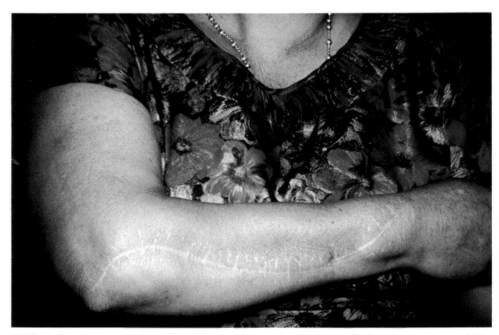

FIG. 4-6. Postoperative view of a patient who had a soft-tissue resection of the dorsal compartment of the forearm for sarcoma. Subsequent tendon transfer procedures will achieve functional rehabilitation after this type of resection.

Soft-Part Resection for Sarcoma of the Anterior Arm

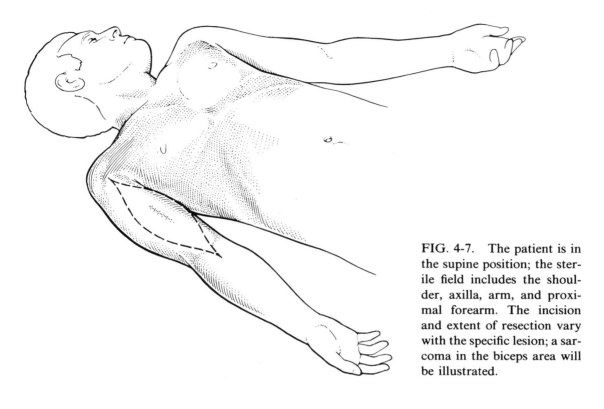

FIG. 4-7. The patient is in the supine position; the sterile field includes the shoulder, axilla, arm, and proximal forearm. The incision and extent of resection vary with the specific lesion; a sarcoma in the biceps area will be illustrated.

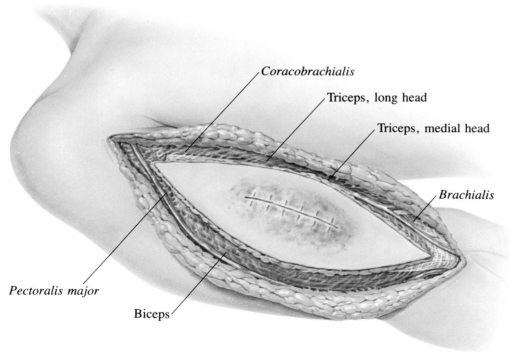

FIG. 4-8. The elliptical incision will generally extend from the deltopectoral groove to the antecubital fossa with adequate skin and subcutaneous tissue around the biopsy site. Medial and lateral flaps are developed until the medial and lateral intermuscular septa are identified. Once the local margins are assured, the level of dissection for these flaps is just superficial to the investing fascia.

53

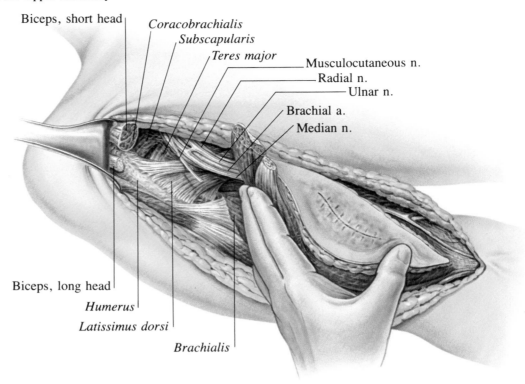

FIG. 4-9.   The long and short head of the biceps and the coracobrachialis are identified proximally and traced under the humeral insertion of the pectoralis major. They are divided just distal to their proximal origins. The musculocutaneous nerve is identified where it approaches the coracobrachialis and is divided. At this point, the neurovascular bundle extending distally from the axilla is identified as these structures enter the medial aspect of the arm between the coracobrachialis and the tendons of latissimus dorsi and teres major. Tumor extension to involve the neurovascular structures will necessitate amputation.

FIG. 4-10.   Once detached from their origins, these muscles (biceps and coracobrachialis) are pulled forward, and dissection proceeds along the medial intermuscular septum toward the humerus. The brachial artery and vein and median and ulnar nerves are identified, traced along the medial compartment of the arm, and retracted from the area of dissection. At this point, the brachialis muscle is identified prior to its dissection from the humerus. Dissection is also carried out laterally along the intermuscular septum in a fashion analogous to that described for the medial dissection.

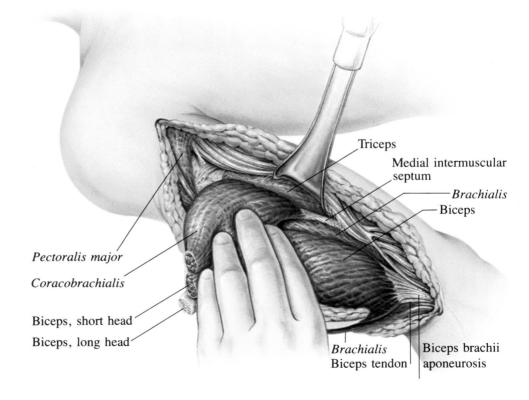

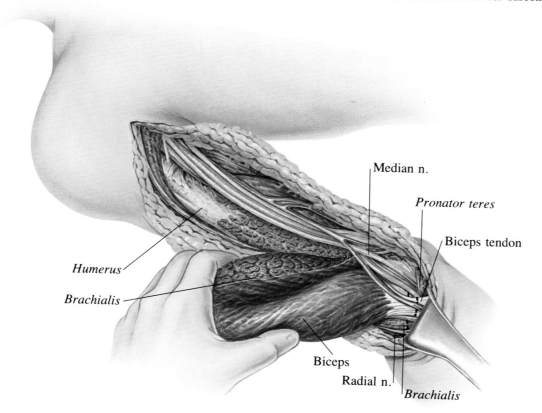

Median n.

Pronator teres

Biceps tendon

Humerus

Brachialis

Biceps

Radial n.

Brachialis

FIG. 4-11. The coracobrachialis and the brachialis are then stripped from the humerus with the help of a periosteal elevator or scalpel. As the dissection approaches the lower third of the arm, the median and radial nerves are exposed as they enter the antecubital fossa from their more medial and posterior arm compartment. At this point, the biceps and brachialis tendons are exposed and cut, and the muscle group is removed.

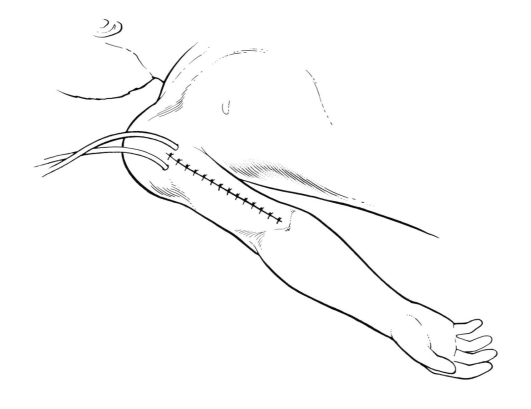

FIG. 4-12. The wound is irrigated, and two catheters for suction are placed along the operative site. The wound is closed in two layers. Major skin defects may require split-thickness skin grafting. Sling immobilization is useful in the early postoperative period. If the radial nerve has been sacrificed, tendon transfers in the forearm will produce an excellent functional result and prevent a wrist drop; nerve grafting is not necessary.

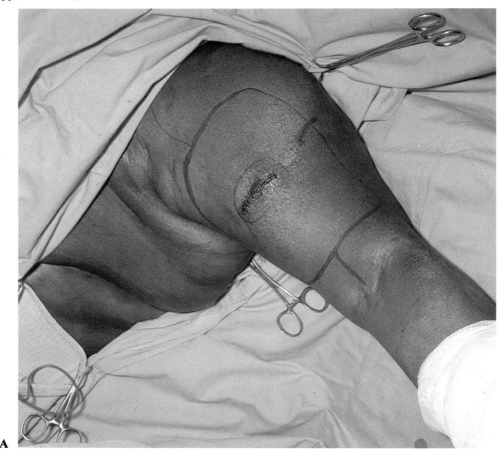

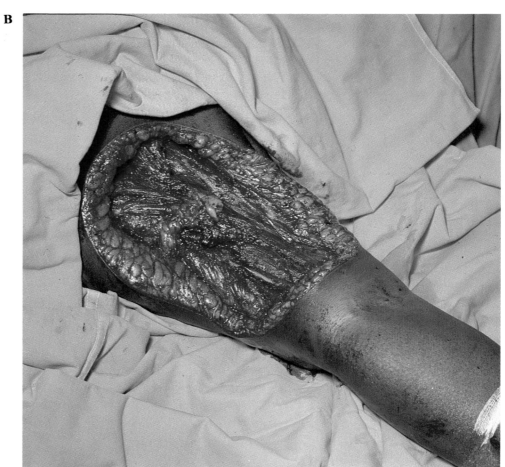

FIG. 4-13. Preoperative (A) and operative (B) views of soft-tissue resection for a small fibrosarcoma arising in the region of the biceps muscle.

56

Soft-Part Resection for Sarcoma of the Posterior Arm

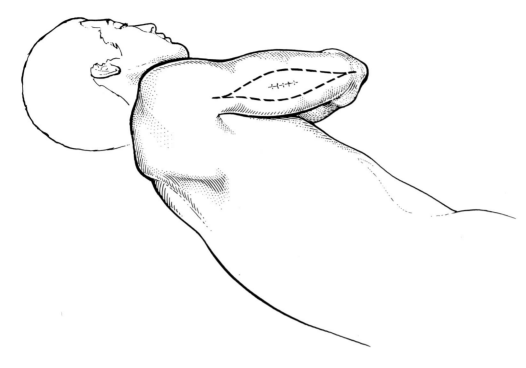

FIG. 4-14. The patient is placed in a semisupine position with the arm lying across the chest. The sterile field includes the shoulder, axilla, arm, and proximal forearm. The skin incision around the biopsy wound is outlined.

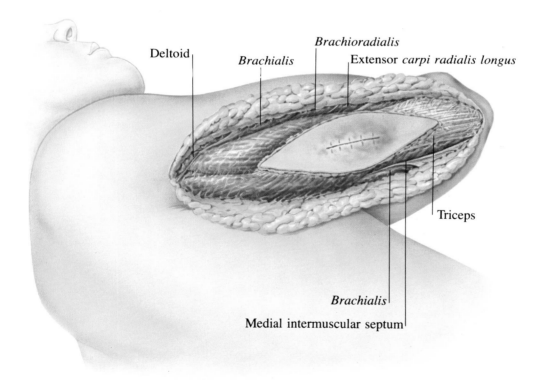

Deltoid · *Brachialis* · *Brachioradialis* · Extensor *carpi radialis longus* · Triceps · *Brachialis* · Medial intermuscular septum

FIG. 4-15. The incision is made along the posterior aspect of the arm extending from the deltoid to a point just proximal to the olecranon for most lesions in this area, but the incision naturally varies depending on the size and position of the neoplasm. Adequate skin and subcutaneous margins are required around the biopsy site. Medial and lateral flaps are developed, external to the investing fascia, until the medial and lateral intermuscular septa are reached.

57

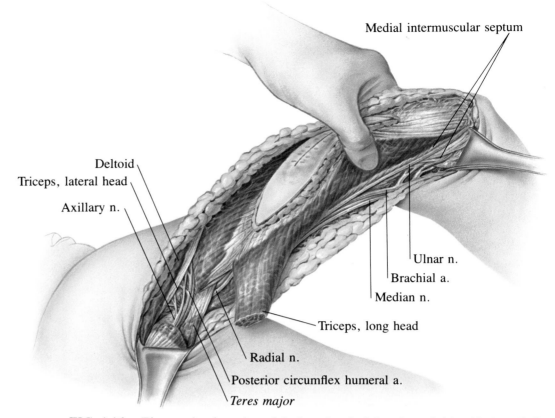

Medial intermuscular septum

Deltoid

Triceps, lateral head

Axillary n.

Ulnar n.

Brachial a.

Median n.

Triceps, long head

Radial n.

Posterior circumflex humeral a.

Teres major

FIG. 4-16. The proximal portion of the long head of the triceps is identified medially, traced under the deltoid toward the scapula, and divided at the point where it crosses the teres major. At this point, the surgeon should identify the axillary and radial nerves and the circumflex artery as they leave the axilla to enter the posterior compartment of the arm. The dissection next extends along the medial intermuscular septum on the surface of the long head of the triceps. The brachial vessels, with the median and ulnar nerves, are exposed and retracted from the area of resection.

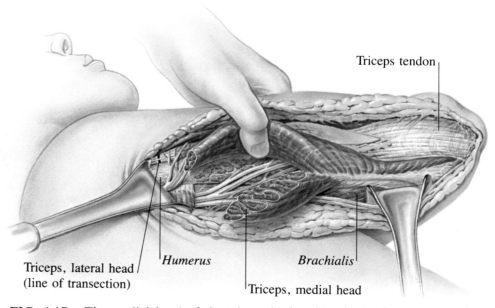

Triceps tendon

Triceps, lateral head
(line of transection)

Humerus

Brachialis

Triceps, medial head

FIG. 4-17. The medial head of the triceps is then identified where it arises from the humerus. With a periosteal elevator, its fibers of origin are stripped from the humerus with care to avoid injury to the radial nerve as it loops around the middle third of the humerus.

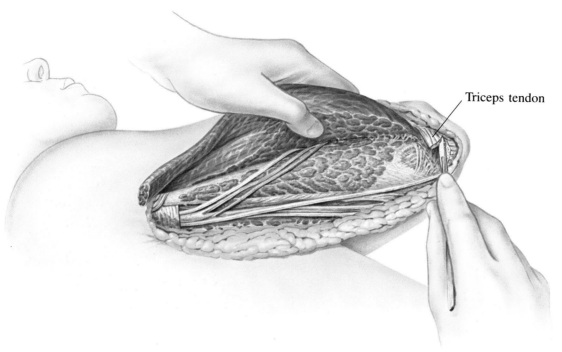

Triceps tendon

FIG. 4-18. With the triceps detached proximally, the dissection is carried toward the elbow, separating the remaining triceps origin from the humerus. If the tumor is in close proximity to the periosteum, a longitudinal segment of bone may be removed with a power saw, but such operative findings may lead to the decision to amputate. The inability to achieve an adequate gross margin around the sarcoma may not be apparent until this point in the operative procedure, but the potential problem is one that should be anticipated. Also, the radial nerve may be sacrificed if it is adherent to or involved by the sarcoma. (If sacrifice of the radial nerve is required, excellent wrist extension can be provided by tendon transfers in the forearm). Upon reaching the elbow, the triceps tendon is divided at the level of the olecranon, and the surgical specimen is removed.

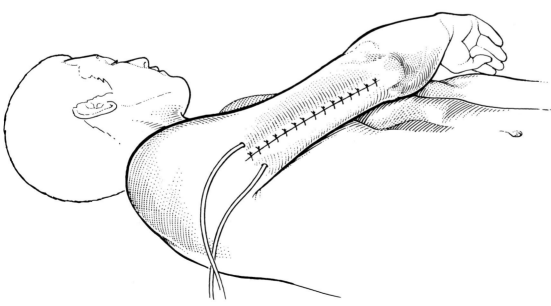

FIG. 4-19. The wound is closed with two layers of interrupted sutures. Suction drainage is useful, and we utilize sling immobilization in the early postoperative period.

59

Scapulectomy for Soft-Part Sarcoma

Total scapulectomy is an infrequently performed operation, primarily utilized for sarcomas arising within the scapula. It is also applicable for soft-tissue tumors overlying the scapula, without chest wall involvement. If the sarcoma extends laterally beyond the confines of the scapula, interscapulothoracic amputation will usually be required. The advantage of scapulectomy is, obviously, the preservation of a functional arm.

The major functional problem following scapulectomy is the loss of abduction of the arm. If the entire trapezius, latissimus dorsi, and deltoid can be preserved, some shoulder abduction will be maintained. With a vigorous physical therapy program, reasonable lower arm function can be restored after this procedure.

References

1. Papaioannou A, Francis K: Scapulectomy for the treatment of primary malignant tumors of the scapula. Clin Orthop 41:125–132, 1965.
2. Ramirez J, Arlen M, Jourdain LM: Total scapulectomy for soft part tumor of the shoulder girdle. Surgery 69:271–275, 1971.

Technique of Scapulectomy

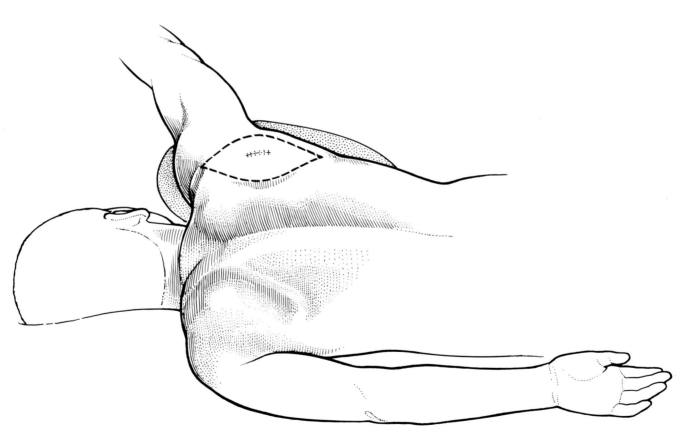

FIG. 4-20. The patient is placed in a semiprone position with the affected side elevated from the operating table, resting over sandbags, to facilitate access to the supraclavicular and axillary regions. The sterile field includes the shoulder, the axilla, and the posterior hemithorax.

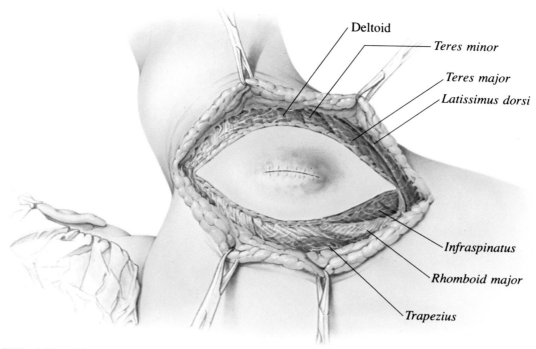

FIG. 4-21. The scapula is approached through a vertical elliptical incision including the biopsy site and the skin overlying the neoplasm. Medial and lateral flaps are developed beyond the anatomic boundaries of the scapula, exposing its muscular attachments.

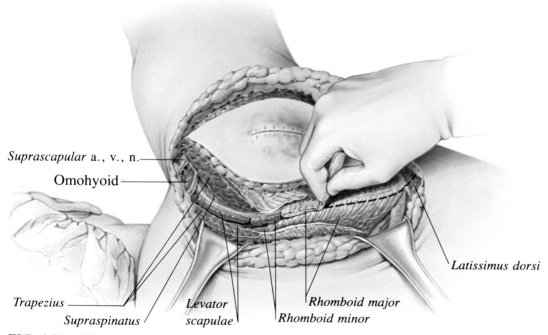

FIG. 4-22. The resection begins by freeing the scapula from its dorsal and cervical muscular attachments. The incision follows the medial border of the scapula, dividing the trapezius, the rhomboids, and the portion of the latissimus dorsi that crosses the lower end of the scapula. As the superior portions of the trapezius and levator scapulae are divided, the transverse cervical vessels and suprascapular vessels and nerve are exposed in the suprascapular region; these vessels are then ligated and divided.

61

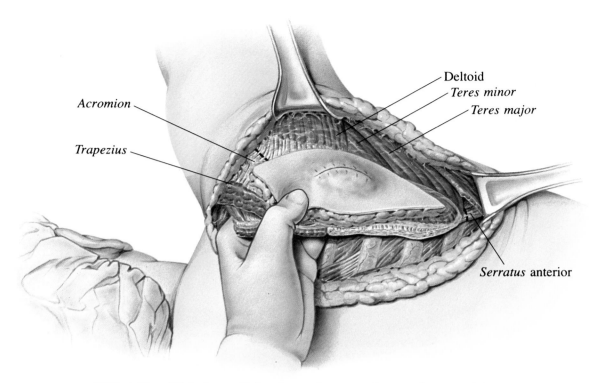

Deltoid
Teres minor
Teres major

Acromion

Trapezius

Serratus anterior

FIG. 4-23.   With the medial and superior muscular attachments divided, the scapula can be retracted laterally by introducing the hand along the chest wall under the scapula and the musculature deep to it. This allows better identification of the lateral border of the scapula. The lateral muscular incision follows this border, and the latissimus dorsi and serratus anterior are divided.

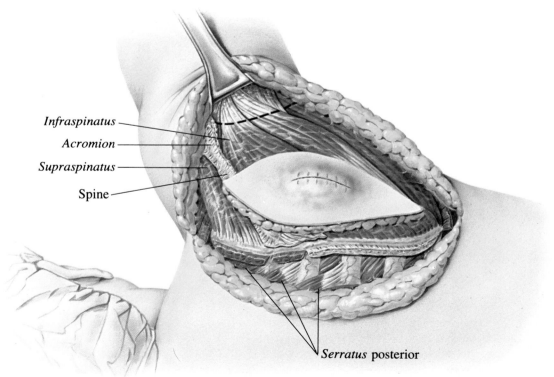

Infraspinatus

Acromion

Supraspinatus

Spine

Serratus posterior

FIG. 4-24.   At this point, the scapula is held in place by muscular attachments to the shoulder joint. The distal humeral insertions of the teres major, teres minor, and supraspinatus are divided. The acromion is then exposed by incising the insertions of the deltoid, trapezius, and supraspinatus muscles on the bony spine of the scapula.

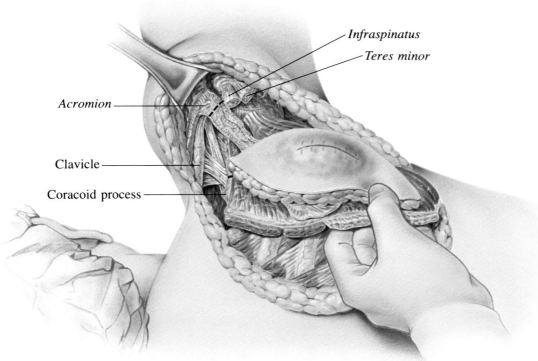

FIG. 4-25.   The acromion is divided with a Gigli saw, preserving the acromioclavicular joint. The coracoid process is then exposed and is severed from the scapula along with its muscular insertions.

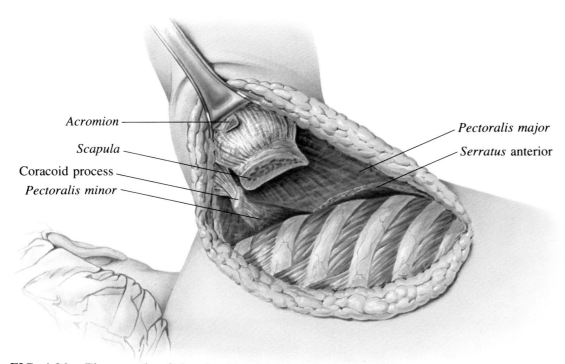

FIG. 4-26.   The capsule of the shoulder joint is now exposed. With a Gigli saw, the scapula is divided proximal to the glenoid fossa, leaving the articular face, ligaments, and joint capsule intact. Retaining the shoulder joint allows normal arm function and reasonable shoulder motion despite the loss of ability to elevate or abduct the upper extremity.

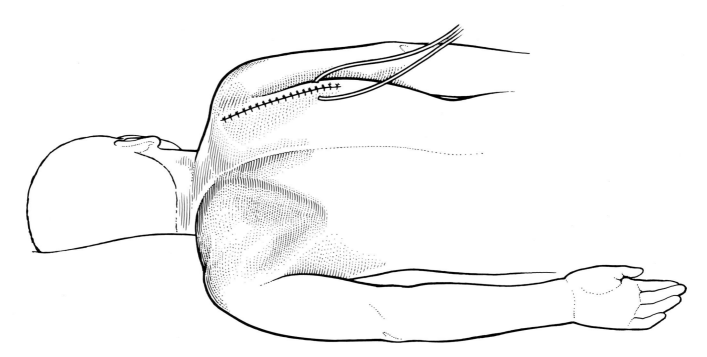

FIG. 4-27. After removal of the surgical specimen the operative wound is irrigated and closed. Suction catheters are employed for drainage, and a Valpeau dressing or sling is utilized for partial immobilization during the early postoperative period. Physical therapy is useful for rehabilitation after the suction catheters have been removed and healing has progressed satisfactorily.

Interscapulothoracic Amputation

Amputation of the entire upper extremity, the shoulder girdle, and its muscular attachments was first termed "interscapulothoracic amputation" in 1887 by the French surgeon Berger (1). There are a number of previous isolated case reports of similar procedures for gunshot wounds, other trauma, and for tumors, but Berger's report standardized the technique that is employed today and recorded an operative mortality of only 10.4%. Although there should be virtually no mortality for interscapulothoracic amputation performed today, the operative mortality for the collected experience prior to Berger's report was 38%! In 1900 Buchanan (3) secured and summarized follow-up information on a total of 141 interscapulothoracic amputations performed prior to that time, but the operation was still rarely employed. By 1942 George Pack and his colleagues (4) at the Memorial Hospital (New York) had culled another 180 cases of this operation performed since 1900; they added 31 cases of their own without a single operative death. In the four decades since this report, interscapulothoracic amputation continues to be an infrequently performed operation. Neoplastic indications are primarily soft-tissue and bone sarcomas that are not anatomically suitable for limb preservation operations.

The indications for interscapulothoracic amputation include malignant tumors that would require disarticulation of the humerus, malignant tumors invading the capsule of the shoulder joint, and neoplasms involving the neurovascular bundle in the axilla. Little is gained by disarticulation of the humerus for sarcomas in the proximal arm that are unsuitable for soft-part resection, since a functional arm prosthesis is not really feasible. For such lesions a better surgical margin is obtained by interscapulothoracic amputation without altering the degree of functional disability. The cosmetic deformity is great, but suitable prostheses for the shoulder deformity are easily made and readily available. They provide a base for proper fit of clothing and an acceptable external appearance.

A difficult problem sometimes presented is the operative choice between soft-part resection and interscapulothoracic amputation in the patient in whom a less than optimal margin is obtained by the lesser procedure even though a clear microscopic margin can be achieved. Radiation is often administered as adjuvant therapy in this situation to increase the opportunity for local disease control. This may be justified despite the lack of prospective controlled trials to establish this as an equal alternative to amputation (see Chapter 11). However, the operative procedure must produce clear margins on pathologic study to ensure local control whether or not radiation is employed.

There are no major variations in the procedure of interscapulothoracic amputation from the standpoint of the extent of resection of bony structures except for that subset of patients that may require resection of an adjacent portion of the chest wall. A minor variation in the standard technique is the disarticulation of the sternoclavicular joint rather than transection of the medial segment of the clavicle (2). This variation is particularly useful when partial or complete neck dissection is performed in conjunction with the amputation. The addition of neck dissection to the procedure would be a consideration for patients with melanoma more than for those with sarcoma. The variations in the extent of soft-tissue resection, and differences in the placement of the surgical incisions, are obviously related to the anatomic location and extent of the individual neoplasms.

Complications of interscapulothoracic amputation are rare and are limited to occasional necrosis or infection of the skin flaps. Rehabilitation of the patient after this operation requires learning to depend on only one arm and hand, since the standard shoulder or arm prostheses employed are nonfunctional and are mainly for cosmesis. The physical rehabilitation team of physiatrist, physical therapist, and occupational therapist can teach such patients to button buttons, dress themselves, and expand one-arm functions to incorporate many tasks previously requiring both upper extremities. Although there are some specific limitations, these patients can be gainfully employed and live essentially normal lives.

References

1. Berger P: L'amputation du membre supérieur dans la contiguité du tronc (amputation interscapulo-thoracique). Paris, G Masson, 1887.
2. Bowden L: A more thorough in-continuity neck and axillary dissection. Ann Surg 143:481–492, 1956.
3. Buchanan JJ: Phila Med J 6:73–82, 1900.
4. Pack GT, McNeer G, Coley BL: Interscapulothoracic amputation for malignant tumors of the upper extremity. Surg Gynecol Obstet 74:161–175, 1942.

Technique of Interscapulothoracic (IST) Amputation

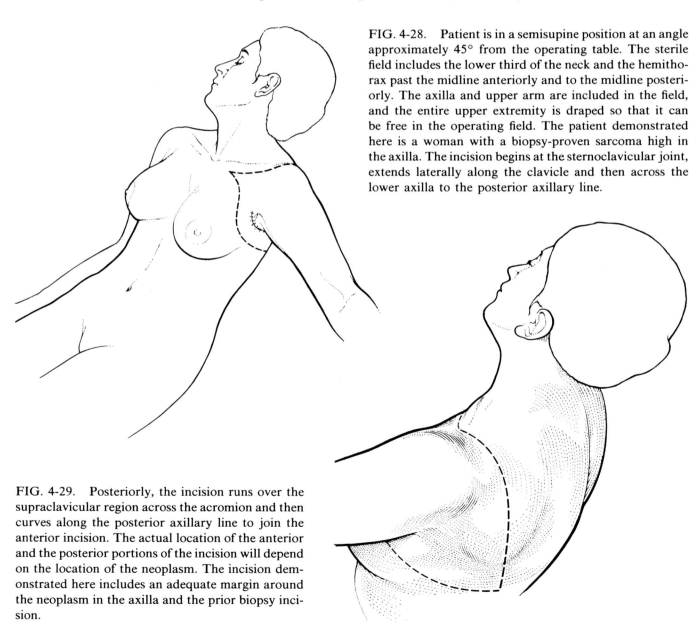

FIG. 4-28.   Patient is in a semisupine position at an angle approximately 45° from the operating table. The sterile field includes the lower third of the neck and the hemithorax past the midline anteriorly and to the midline posteriorly. The axilla and upper arm are included in the field, and the entire upper extremity is draped so that it can be free in the operating field. The patient demonstrated here is a woman with a biopsy-proven sarcoma high in the axilla. The incision begins at the sternoclavicular joint, extends laterally along the clavicle and then across the lower axilla to the posterior axillary line.

FIG. 4-29.   Posteriorly, the incision runs over the supraclavicular region across the acromion and then curves along the posterior axillary line to join the anterior incision. The actual location of the anterior and the posterior portions of the incision will depend on the location of the neoplasm. The incision demonstrated here includes an adequate margin around the neoplasm in the axilla and the prior biopsy incision.

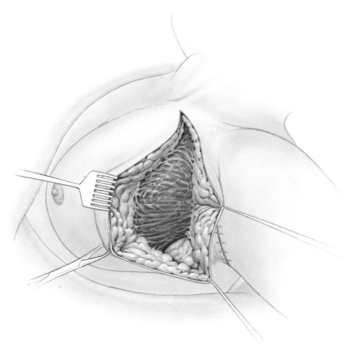

FIG. 4-30. The initial and major part of the dissection is carried out anteriorly. Dissection is at the fascial level over the pectoralis major.

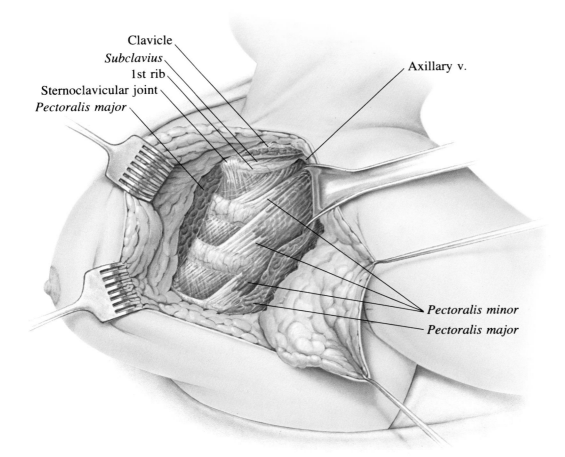

FIG. 4-31. The pectoralis major is divided on the anterior chest wall after it is exposed by means of mobilizing the anterior skin flap. The pectoralis minor is exposed, as well as the axillary vein just beyond the first rib.

67

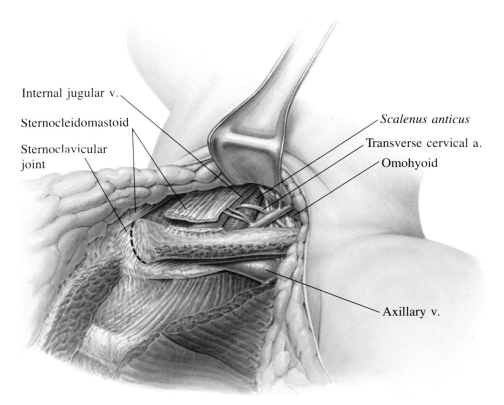

Internal jugular v.

Sternocleidomastoid

Sternoclavicular joint

Scalenus anticus

Transverse cervical a.

Omohyoid

Axillary v.

FIG. 4-32. The site of origin of the sternocleidomastoid on the medial aspect of the clavicle is divided prior to opening the sternoclavicular joint. Care is taken to avoid injury to the structures in the carotid sheath. The dotted line is the site for opening the joint anteriorly.

FIG. 4-33. The sternoclavicular ligaments in the region of the sternoclavicular joint have been divided, and the head of the clavicle has been disarticulated at the level of this joint. Care is necessary during division of the posterior capsule of this joint to avoid injury to the underlying innominate vein. The juncture of the subclavian and jugular veins to form the innominate vein is well exposed by this disarticulation.

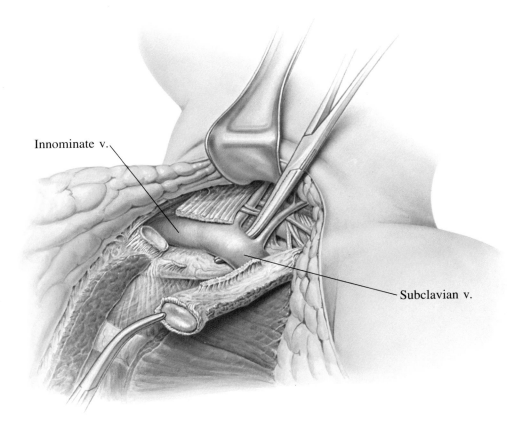

Innominate v.

Subclavian v.

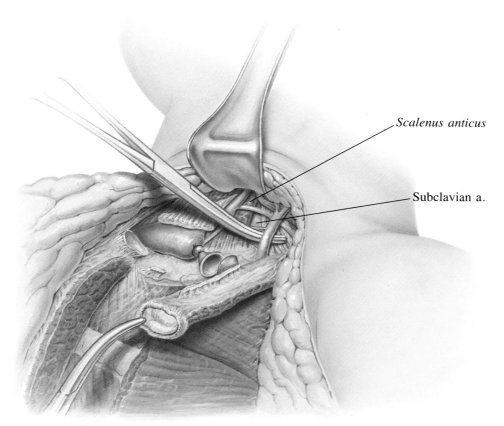

Scalenus anticus

Subclavian a.

FIG. 4-34. The remaining attachments of the clavicle in the region of the sternoclavicular joint have been divided, along with the subclavius muscle, and the arm is rotated laterally to allow this lateral retraction of the head of the clavicle. This exposes the innominate vein, the internal jugular vein, and the junction of the internal jugular and subclavian veins on the scalenus anticus. The subclavian vein is isolated in preparation for later ligation, but innominate vein ligation is appropriate if the procedure is carried out in a situation where neck dissection is advisable (e.g., selected instances for melanoma). This option is rarely indicated for sarcomas.

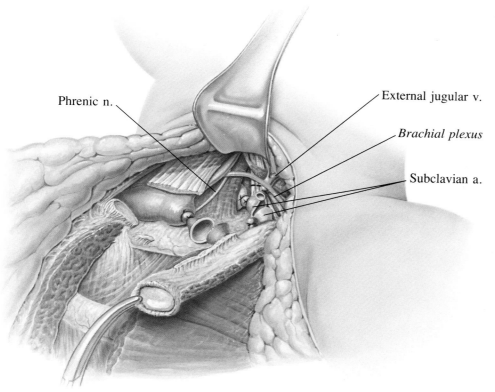

Phrenic n.

External jugular v.

Brachial plexus

Subclavian a.

FIG. 4-35. Dissection is deepened laterally along the scalenus anticus to its lateral border, where the subclavian artery is exposed coming from behind the muscle. The artery is isolated, ligated, and suture-ligated at this point. When this is accomplished, the subclavian vein is ligated, divided, and suture-ligated. These ligations have been completed in the drawing. The major structures that remain are the cords of the brachial plexus. The trunks of the brachial plexus are exposed and divided sharply with a knife at the level indicated. The areolar tissue in the axilla is then swept laterally from the chest wall to the subscapular muscle, and this completes the anterior portion of the dissection.

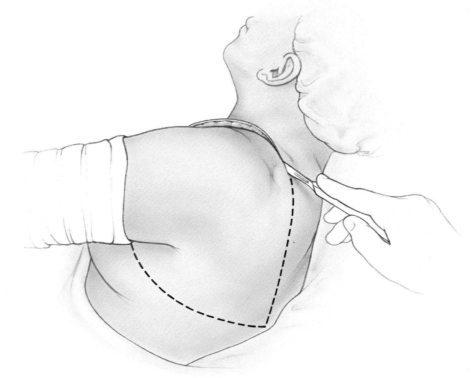

FIG. 4-36. The upper extremity is now rotated medially, and the posterior skin incision is made. Dissection of the posterior skin flap is carried out at the level of the muscle fascia, thereby exposing the broad muscle attachment of the trapezius and the latissimus dorsi.

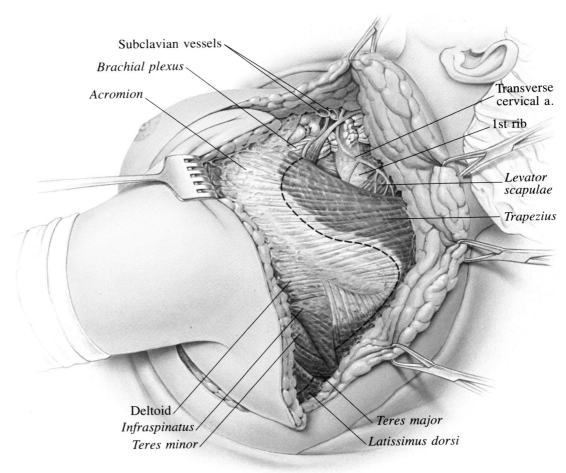

FIG. 4-37. The remaining muscle attachments are posterior and medial to the scapula. The trapezius and latissimus dorsi are divided, exposing the deeper musculature.

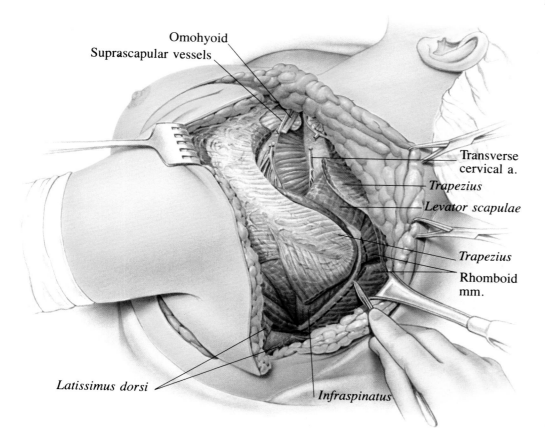

Omohyoid
Suprascapular vessels

Transverse
cervical a.
Trapezius
Levator scapulae

Trapezius
Rhomboid
mm.

Latissimus dorsi

Infraspinatus

FIG. 4-38. The levator scapulae and rhomboid muscles are next divided along with the suprascapular vessels and the transverse cervical artery. Transection of the pectoralis minor and the serratus anterior completes the posterior dissection, and the operative specimen is removed.

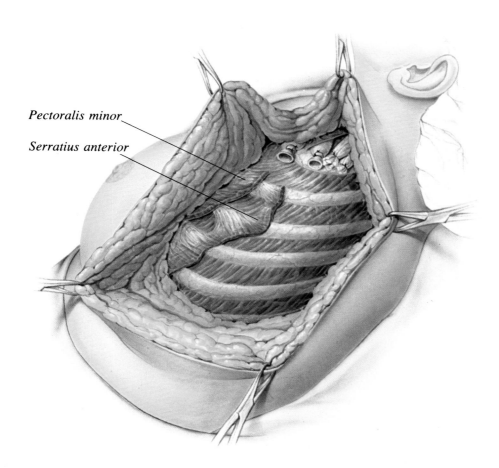

Pectoralis minor

Serratius anterior

FIG. 4-39. The operative field after the radical amputation has been completed. The transected major artery, vein, and brachial plexus are seen along with the ribs and intercostal muscles of the chest wall.

71

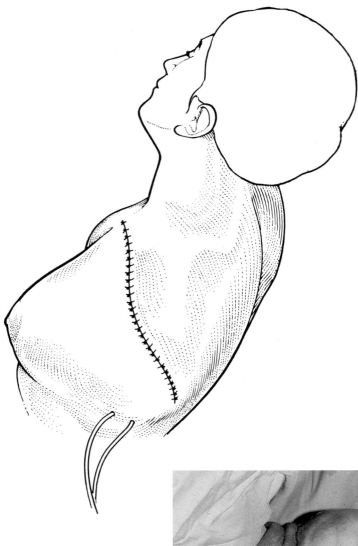

FIG. 4-40. The wound is closed with suction drains using subcutaneous and skin closure after trimming off excess skin and subcutaneous tissue.

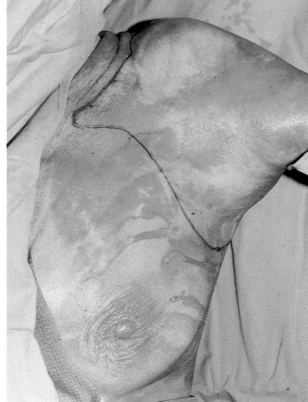

FIG. 4-41. Operative views of interscapulothoracic amputation. The incision is outlined for this malignant mesenchymoma in the axillary region of a 65-year-old female (**A**). (*Continued*)

A

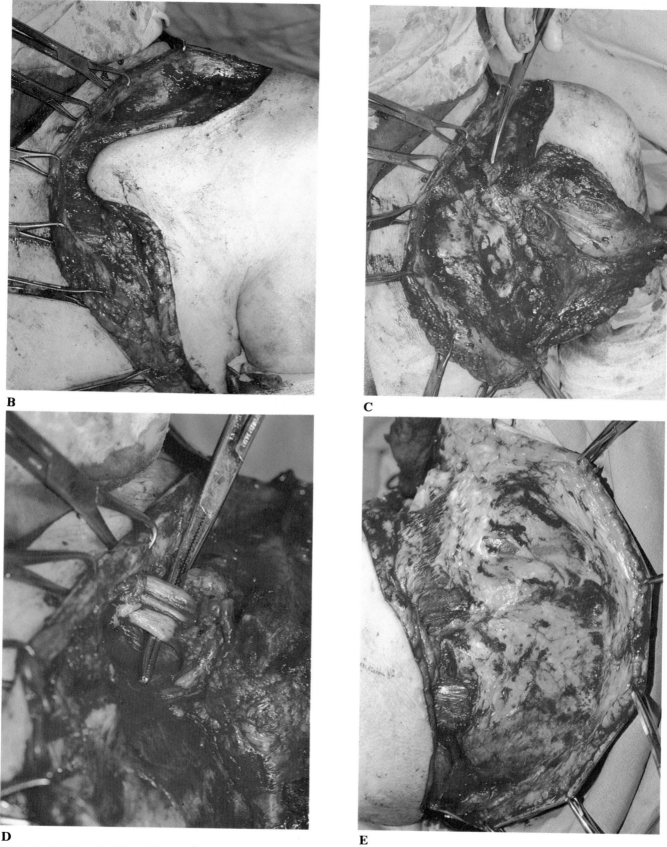

B

C

D

E

FIG. 4-41 (*Cont.*)   The skin flaps are developed to expose the pectoralis major and the clavicle (**B**). The sternoclavicular joint is opened and disarticulation accomplished (**C**) in preparation for exposure of the neurovascular bundle, which is demonstrated in **D**. The posterior skin flap is dissected, exposing the musculature over the scapula (**E**). (*Continued*)

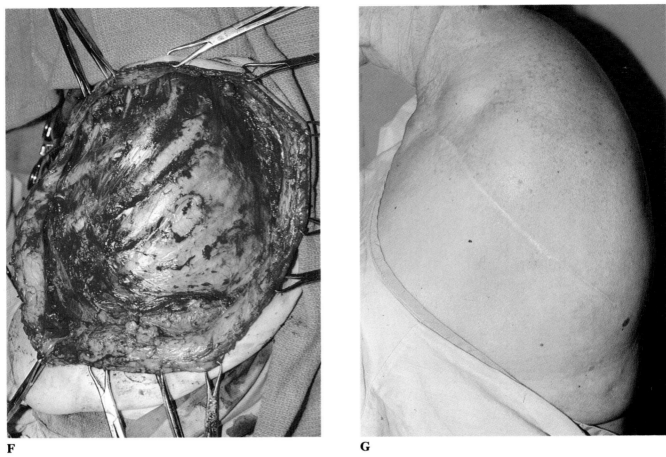

F

G

FIG. 4-41. (*Cont.*) The completed amputation field is seen in **F** prior to primary closure of the wound. The healed amputation site is shown in **G**.

Operations for Sarcomas on the Lower Extremity

5

From the standpoint of choice of operative procedure, it is fortunate that the thigh is one of the more frequent sites of origin of soft-tissue sarcomas. Both the anatomy and bulk of tissue in this site often allow an adequate soft-part resection in terms of tumor margin, and "limb salvage" can be achieved. It is also possible in many instances to obtain an adequate local margin around the sarcoma by wide but intracompartmental excision. However, the size of the sarcoma and the nonfunctional nature of the musculature proximal and distal to the muscle resection usually lead to essentially total compartmental resection. The choice of patients for amputation is made on an anatomic basis, with standard operative techniques being employed except for proximal thigh and buttock lesions. The technique of hemipelvectomy or hip joint disarticulation is utilized if amputation is required.

Soft-Part Resection for Sarcoma of the Anterior Thigh (Quadriceps)

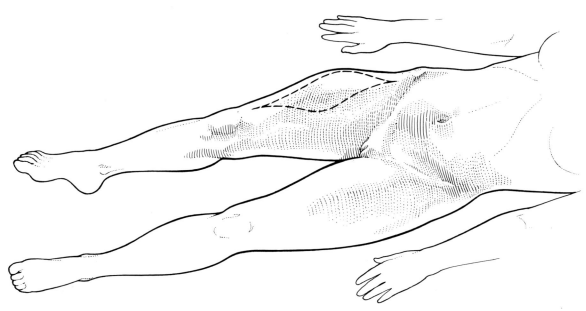

FIG. 5-1. The entire thigh is prepped circumferentially and draped from the inguinal area to a point just below the knee. A wide ellipse of skin is outlined by an incision designed to encompass all possible subcutaneous extensions of the underlying sarcoma, as well as the biopsy wound. The specific location and extent of skin resection depends on the individual presentation.

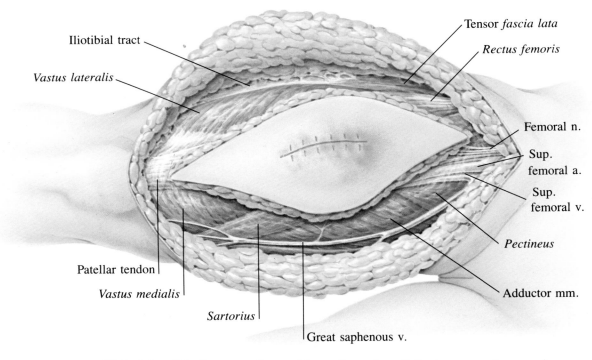

FIG. 5-2. Skin flaps are dissected laterally and medially to expose the muscle mass to be resected. The flaps are dissected just above the fascial layer that covers the quadriceps and adductor muscles. The gracilis is seen at the medial extent of dissection and the tensor fascia lata laterally. Adequate resection of the skin over the neoplasm obviates the need for thin skin flaps during this portion of the dissection.

76

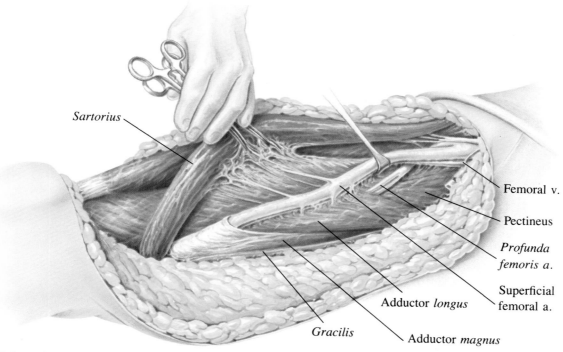

Sartorius

Femoral v.

Pectineus

Profunda femoris a.

Superficial femoral a.

Adductor *longus*

Gracilis

Adductor *magnus*

FIG. 5-3. The next step in the procedure is dissection and mobilization of the femoral vessels from the level of the inguinal ligament distally. The sartorius is shown retracted laterally, and the division of the femoral sheath over the femoral artery and femoral vein exposes these vessels in the proximal anterior thigh.

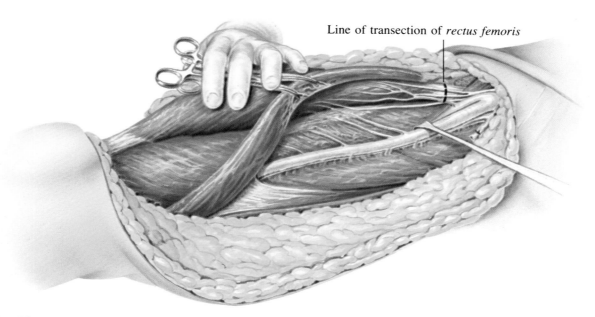

Line of transection of *rectus femoris*

FIG. 5-4. The findings at the time of mobilization of the femoral artery determine whether an adequate margin of normal muscle and fascia around the sarcoma can be achieved. If an adequate margin cannot be achieved, this procedure may need to be aborted and amputation carried out. In this patient, the vessels are freed successfully from the adjacent musculature, thus encompassing the neoplasm from the level of the inguinal ligament proximally to the adductor canal distally. The femoral nerve branches lateral to the femoral vessels are seen. The proximal tendon of the sartorius has been transected.

77

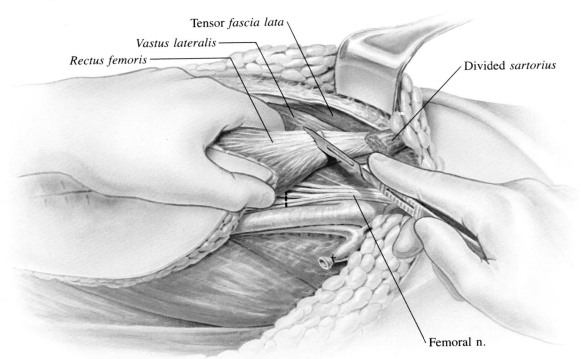

Tensor *fascia lata*

Vastus lateralis

Rectus femoris

Divided *sartorius*

Femoral n.

FIG. 5-5. Resection of the sarcoma is now accomplished by dividing the muscle mass containing or surrounding the neoplasm. Great care is taken to achieve a wide gross margin. The resection does not really require resection of the entire muscle mass from origin to insertion, but this is the most practical approach for these muscles when resection of their midportion is required. Transection of the proximal quadriceps is being accomplished in this view.

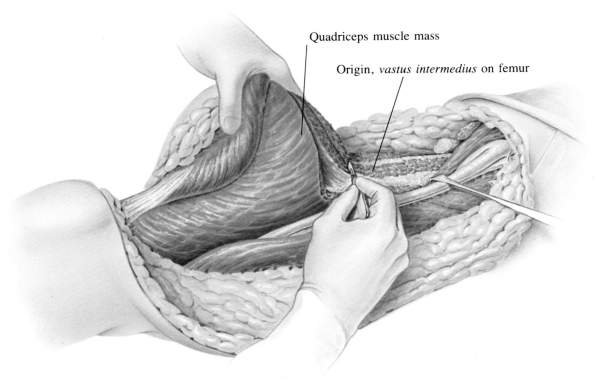

Quadriceps muscle mass

Origin, *vastus intermedius* on femur

FIG. 5-6. The muscle mass containing the neoplasm is dissected distally. The femoral nerve branches to this muscle mass are divided in this process, and the vastus intermedius is divided at its origin from the femur.

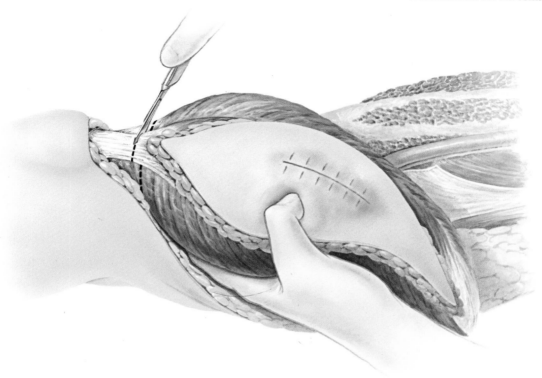

FIG. 5-7. The resection is completed by dividing the distal portion of the patellar tendon and the insertions of the vastus muscles medial and lateral to this at a level high enough to avoid entry into the knee joint (if the joint cavity is entered, it is closed with interrupted sutures).

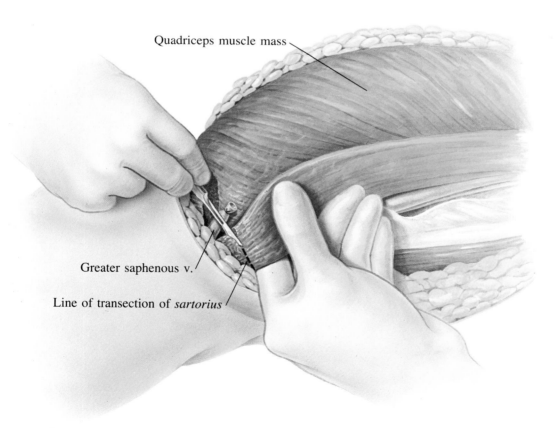

Quadriceps muscle mass

Greater saphenous v.

Line of transection of *sartorius*

FIG. 5-8. The distal sartorius muscle is divided and the specimen is removed.

79

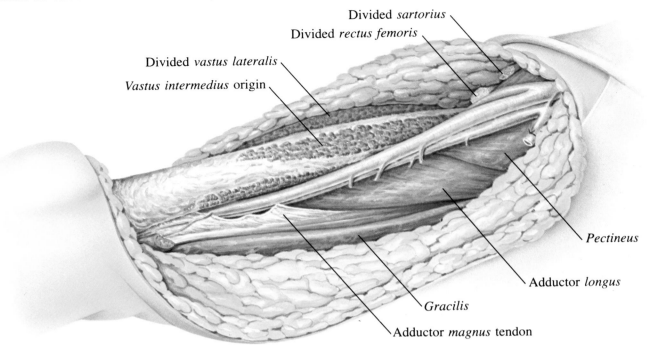

Divided *sartorius*
Divided *rectus femoris*
Divided *vastus lateralis*
Vastus intermedius origin
Pectineus
Adductor *longus*
Gracilis
Adductor *magnus* tendon

FIG. 5-9. The completed dissection shows the exposed femur, the femoral vessels and adductor muscles medially, with a portion of the vastus lateralis at the lateral margin of the dissection.

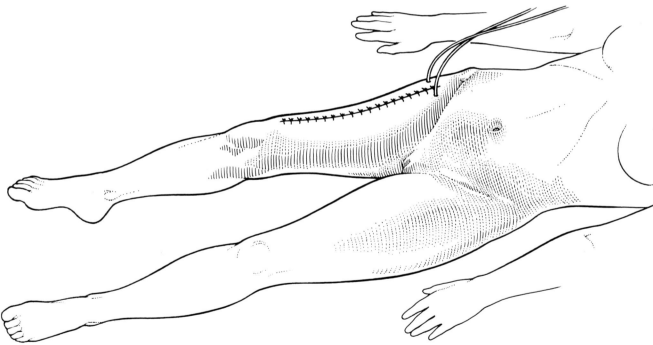

FIG. 5-10. After hemostasis is accomplished, large suction catheters are inserted and the wound is closed by approximation of the skin flaps. Physical therapy is begun on the first postoperative day and starts as active and passive leg-raising exercises. When the suction catheters have been removed walking is begun; initially, this is with a walker or crutches, but most patients rapidly discard these and require no assistance. Despite the loss of the entire quadriceps, most patients are able to walk stairs without difficulty after recovery.

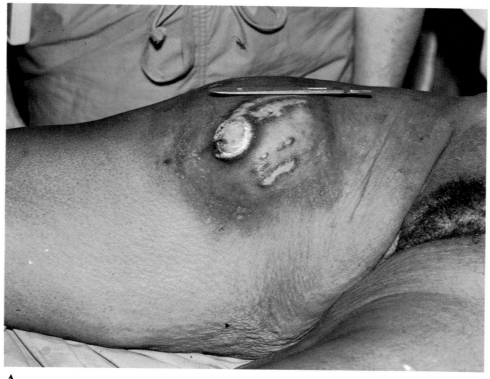

A

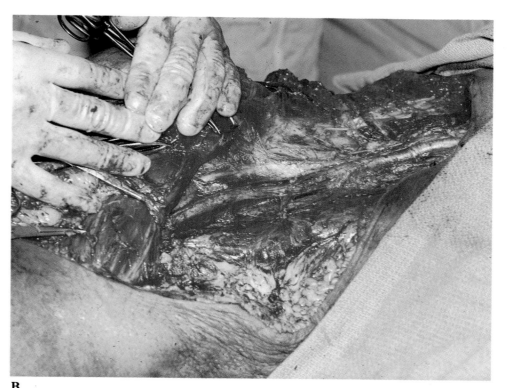

B

FIG. 5-11. Liposarcoma of anterior thigh (quadriceps muscles) eroding through the overlying skin (**A**). Resection of the muscle compartment of the anterior thigh is feasible, due to ability to achieve an adequate soft-tissue margin (**B**). This view demonstrates dissection of the quadriceps and sartorius muscle mass from the femoral vessels.

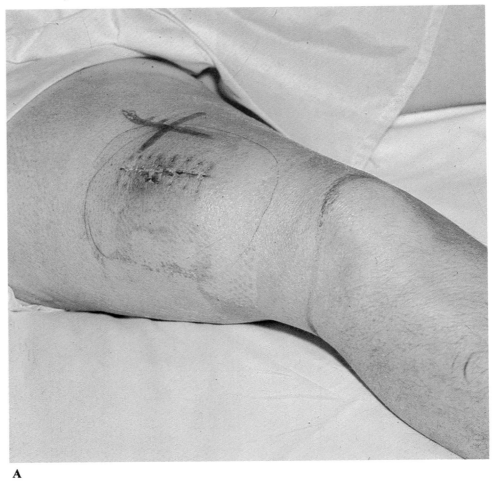

A

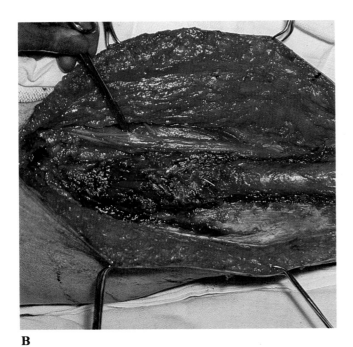

B

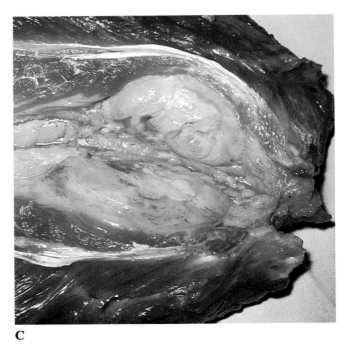

C

FIG. 5-12. Liposarcoma of quadriceps region demonstrating recent biopsy incision and outline of area planned for excision of overlying skin (**A**). Operative field after completion of compartmental resection of quadriceps and sartorius muscles (**B**). The femoral vessels and the femur are seen. Dissected surgical specimen demonstrates the sarcoma contained within the resected muscle mass (**C**).

Soft-Part Resection for Sarcoma in Posterior Thigh Region (Hamstring)

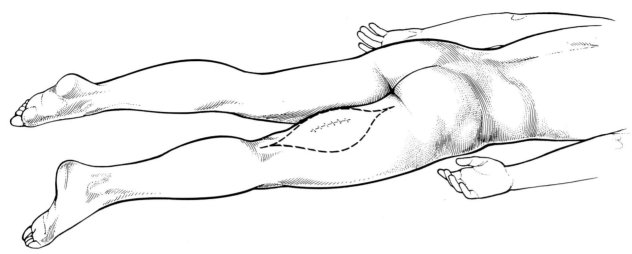

FIG. 5-13. The thigh is prepped and draped circumferentially from the region of the buttock to a level just below the knee. The patient may be placed in the prone position, but a lateral position may be employed if an amputation is considered a possibility prior to the dissection to determine adequacy of the deep margin. An ellipse of skin is outlined over the mass so as to include the entire biopsy wound and all superficial tissues near the sarcoma itself. Transverse extensions of the incision at the level of the infragluteal crease and just above the popliteal space may be used to facilitate development of skin flaps.

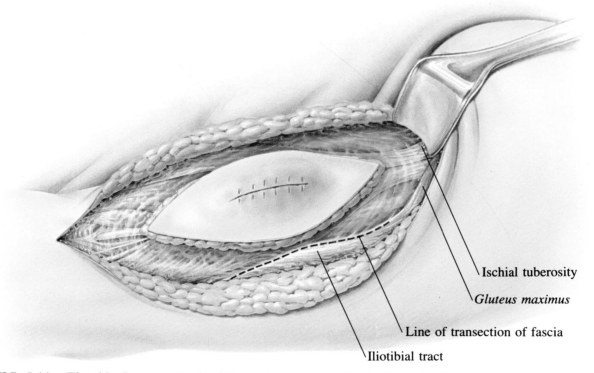

Ischial tuberosity

Gluteus maximus

Line of transection of fascia

Iliotibial tract

FIG. 5-14. The skin flaps are developed in a plane just outside the investing fascia of the musculature of the posterior thigh. The medial extent of dissection is just posterior to the gracilis, and the lateral extent is over the region of the iliotibial tract.

83

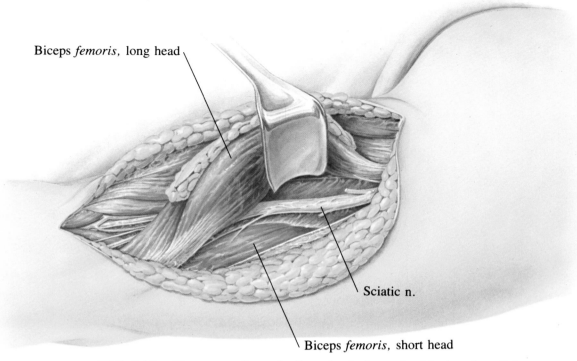

Biceps *femoris,* long head

Sciatic n.

Biceps *femoris,* short head

FIG. 5-15. The extent of muscle dissection is determined by location of the sarcoma, but resection usually includes the three hamstring muscles (long head of the biceps femoris, semimembranosus, and semitendinosus). These are superficial (posterior) to the sciatic nerve and their origin is from the ischial tuberosity. Resection of a sarcoma in this region depends on developing a plane free of neoplasm anterior (deep) to the muscle mass, since the next structure of concern in this region is the sciatic nerve itself.

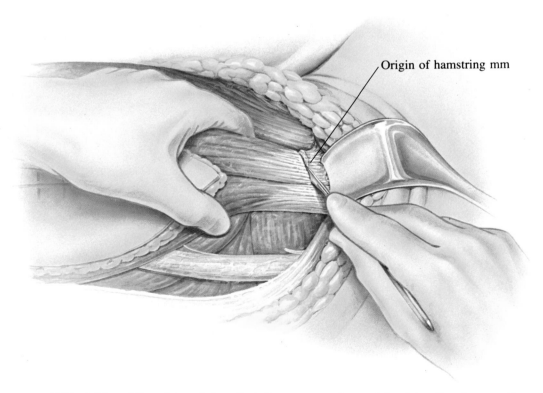

Origin of hamstring mm

FIG. 5-16. After determining that the sarcoma is contained by the deep surface of the hamstring muscle group, their origins are divided just below the ischial tuberosity, exposing the underlying adductor muscle mass.

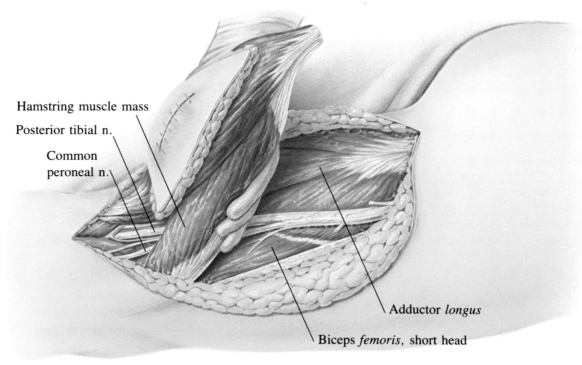

Hamstring muscle mass

Posterior tibial n.

Common
peroneal n.

Adductor *longus*

Biceps *femoris,* short head

FIG. 5-17. The hamstring muscle mass is dissected distally, thereby exposing the adductors and the sciatic nerve as far as the superior portion of the popliteal space. Here the sciatic nerve has divided to form the posterior tibial nerve and the common peroneal nerve.

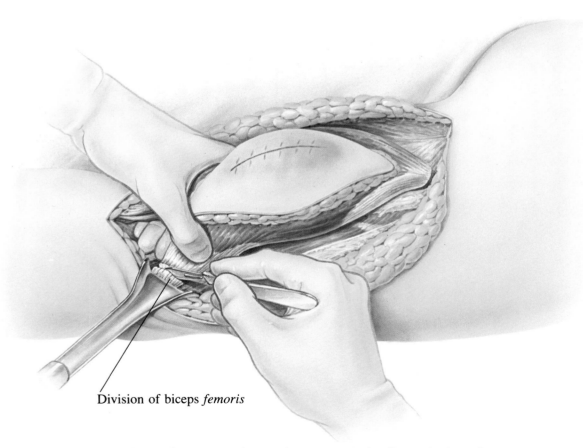

Division of biceps *femoris*

FIG. 5-18. The long head of the biceps femoris is transected distally on the lateral side of the distal thigh, taking care to avoid injury to the common peroneal nerve.

85

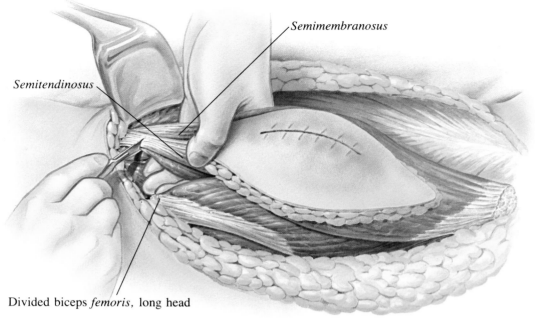

Semimembranosus

Semitendinosus

Divided biceps *femoris,* long head

FIG. 5-19.   The insertions of the semimembranosus and semitendinosus are then divided just above the popliteal space, exposing the medial head of the gastrocnemius muscle.

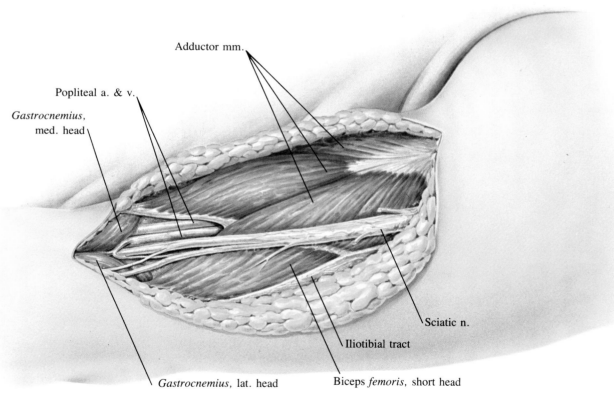

Adductor mm.

Popliteal a. & v.

Gastrocnemius, med. head

Sciatic n.

Iliotibial tract

Gastrocnemius, lat. head

Biceps *femoris,* short head

FIG. 5-20.   The deep plane of the dissection of the hamstrings is completed, and the muscle mass containing the sarcoma and overlying skin is removed. The operative field shows the adductors, the popliteal vessels extending distally, and the short head of the biceps femoris muscle lateral to and behind the sciatic nerve. With a sarcoma impinging on the common peroneal nerve, this branch may be included in the resection and an appropriate splint applied after wound closure.

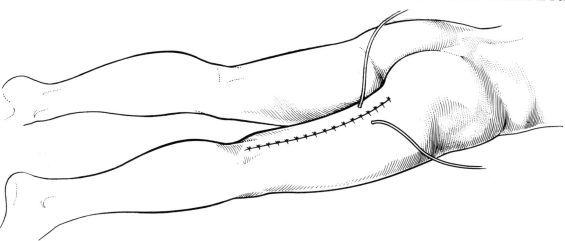

FIG. 5-21. After hemostasis is obtained, suction catheters are inserted and the wound is closed in two layers. Rehabilitation is accomplished in the same fashion as described for resections of the anterior thigh.

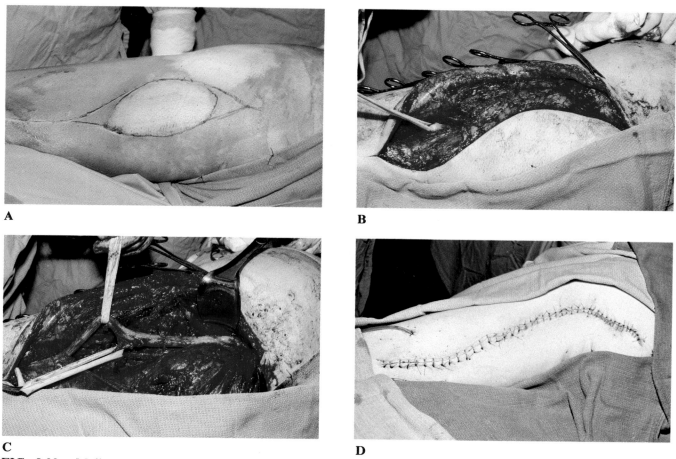

A

B

C

D

FIG. 5-22. Malignant fibrous histiocytoma arising in the posterior thigh showing plan for skin resection around the biopsy site (**A**). Operative dissection over the hamstring muscle group demonstrating the lateral skin flap and preparation for resection of hamstring muscle mass containing the sarcoma (**B**). The common peroneal nerve has been isolated distally. The hamstring muscles with the enclosed sarcoma have been dissected away from the underlying sciatic nerve after it was determined that there was a clear tumor-free margin on this nerve and its branches (**C**). The soft-tissue resection has been completed and primary closure achieved (**D**).

Soft-Part Resection of a Sarcoma Involving the Calf Musculature (Gastrocnemius and Soleus)

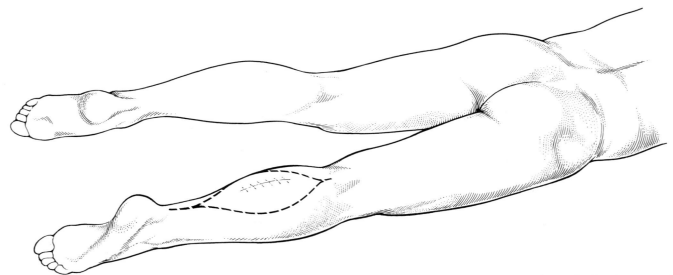

FIG. 5-23. With the patient in a lateral or prone position, the entire leg is prepped circumferentially and draped from a point just above the knee to the ankle. An incision is outlined to adequately encompass the biopsy wound over the calf and achieve an adequate margin over the underlying sarcoma. The breadth of excision should be generous and is tailored to meet the requirements of the specific lesion.

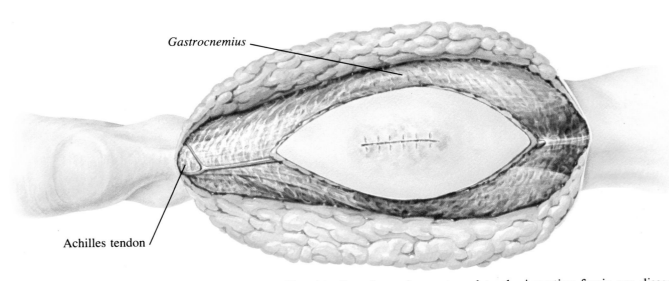

Gastrocnemius

Achilles tendon

FIG. 5-24. The skin flaps in a plane external to the investing fascia are dissected medially to the tibia and laterally to the region of the fibula; this exposes the entire gastrocnemius from the popliteal space to the Achilles tendon.

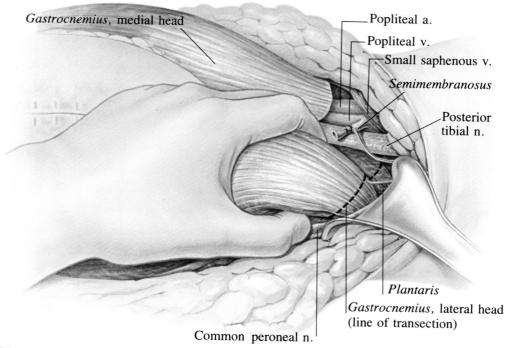

Gastrocnemius, medial head

Popliteal a.

Popliteal v.

Small saphenous v.

Semimembranosus

Posterior
tibial n.

Plantaris

Gastrocnemius, lateral head
(line of transection)

Common peroneal n.

FIG. 5-25.   The medial and lateral heads of the gastrocnemius muscle and the plantaris muscle are divided proximally, with care taken to laterally retract and preserve the laterally situated common peroneal nerve, if this is feasible. The posterior tibial nerve and popliteal vessels are exposed in the depth of the wound.

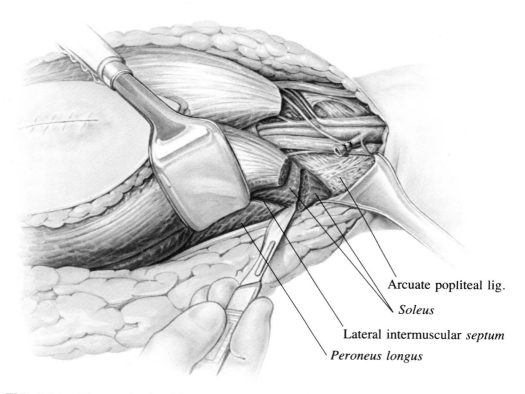

Arcuate popliteal lig.

Soleus

Lateral intermuscular *septum*

Peroneus longus

FIG. 5-26.   The proximal origin of the soleus is next divided and retracted medially, thereby exposing the fibula, the posterior peroneal septum, and the posterior tibial vessels and nerve.

89

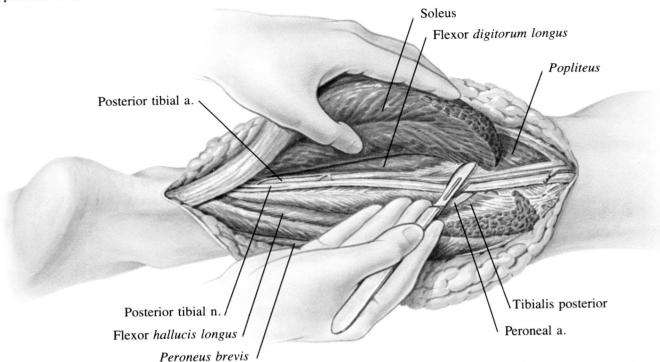

Soleus

Flexor *digitorum longus*

Popliteus

Posterior tibial a.

Posterior tibial n.

Flexor *hallucis longus*

Peroneus brevis

Tibialis posterior

Peroneal a.

FIG. 5-27. The medial dissection separates the soleus from the flexor digitorum longus and allows distal mobilization of the specimen from the underlying structures. The muscle mass encompassing the neoplasm is then dissected distally, exposing and preserving the posterior tibial nerve and vessels lying on the posterior tibialis. This is the ideal plane for dissection if there is an adequate deep margin around the neoplasm, since flexion of the foot will be maintained despite loss of the overlying calf musculature.

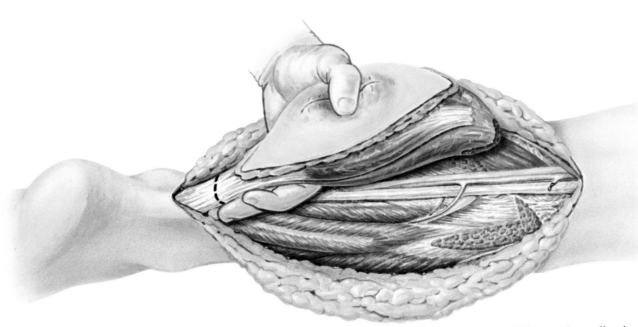

FIG. 5-28. Distally, the specimen is divided through the Achilles tendon, allowing removal of the neoplasm and its surrounding musculature.

90

Tibia

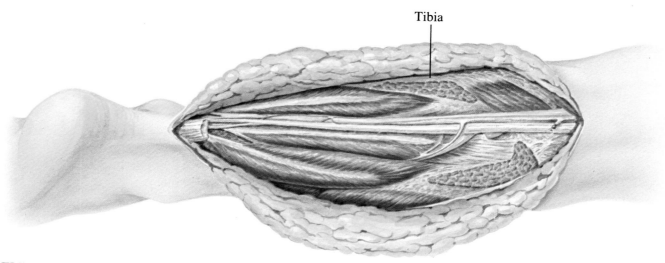

FIG. 5-29. Hemostasis has been obtained in the operative field and the completed dissection is seen. Preservation of the posterior tibial vessels and nerve as shown is a key to this dissection and subsequent rehabilitation of the patient.

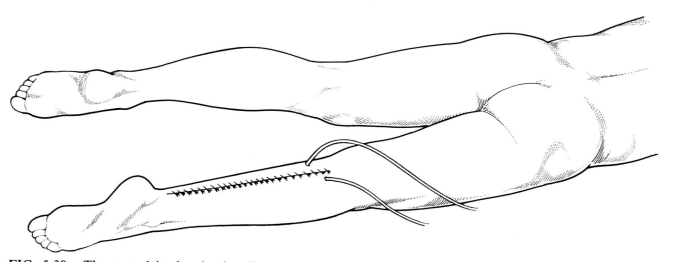

FIG. 5-30. The wound is closed primarily or by means of a long double-pedicle skin flap with a laterally placed split-thickness graft. Suction catheters are employed.

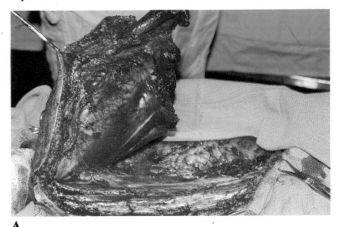

A

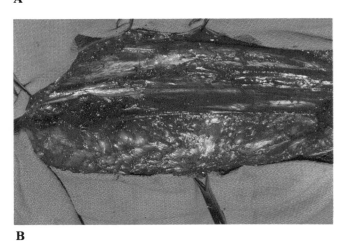

B

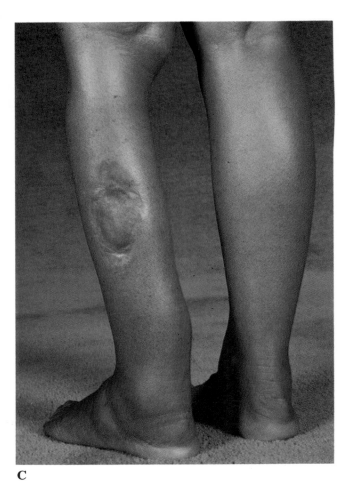

C

FIG. 5-31. A liposarcoma arising from within the calf musculature and contained by the soleus muscle has been found to have a clear soft-tissue margin at the level of the posterior muscle, vessels, and nerve. This overlying muscle compartment is being resected by dissection along this plane (**A**). The operative field at completion of the resection shows the neurovascular structures and the posterior tibialis muscle in the depth of the wound (**B**). The calf deformity from this resection is considerable, but the hypertrophied remaining posterior tibial muscle allows almost normal function (**C**).

Soft-Part Resection of Sarcoma Arising in the Buttock

Resection of the buttock, thus preserving the lower limb, is indicated for sarcomas arising within and confined to the region of the gluteal musculature. Such tumors can be encompassed by a radical resection of the gluteal musculature and overlying soft tissue. Tumors that arise within the buttock and extend beyond the gluteal muscles, thus involving the sciatic nerve, rectum, or adjacent bone, are not candidates for such a procedure because of the very high local recurrence rate, even with adjuvant radiation therapy. Rehabilitation following buttock resections primarily consists of a padded pillow below the resected buttock.

References

1. Bowden L, Booher RJ: Surgical considerations in the treatment of sarcoma of the buttock. Cancer 6:89–99, 1953.
2. Gerson R, Shiu MH, Hajdu SI: Sarcoma of the buttock: a trend toward limb-saving resection. J Surg Oncol 19:238–242, 1982.
3. Sugarbaker PH, Chretien PA: A surgical technique for buttockectomy. Surgery 91:104–107, 1982.
4. Wanebo HJ, Shah J, Knapper W, Hajdu SI, Booher R: Reappraisal of surgical management of sarcoma of the buttock. Cancer 31:97–104, 1973.

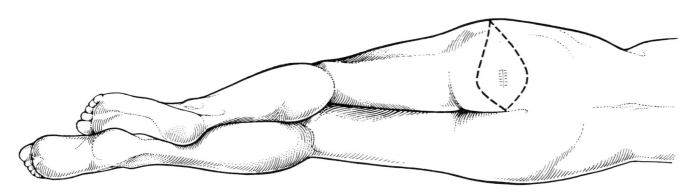

FIG. 5-32.   After applying a temporary purse-string suture around the anus, the patient is prepped over the buttock, lower lumbar region, lower abdomen, and proximal thigh anteriorly and posteriorly. The optimal position is a lateral one to allow the preparation described and allow repositioning of the patient if it is determined during the operation that hemipelvectomy will be required due to depth of invasion of the sarcoma. This is an alternative that must be considered if the deep margin of resection appears inadequate as the operation proceeds. A large ellipse of skin is outlined over the buttock mass as demonstrated here. The extent of skin and subcutaneous resection should encompass the entire operative wound used for biopsy as well as adequate margins around the superficial portion of the neoplasm itself. The medial extent of skin excision is the region of the midline over the sacrum, and the lateral extent is over the greater trochanter of the femur. Variations in the anatomic site of the sarcoma will lead to some minor differences in incision placement.

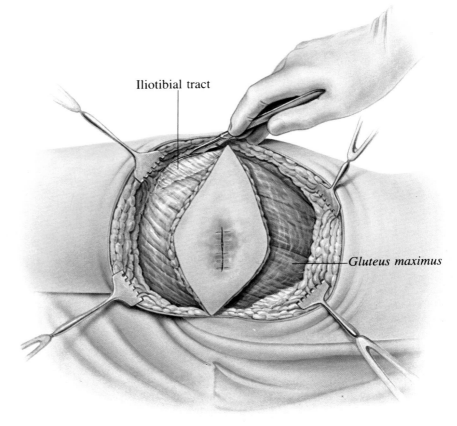

FIG. 5-33. The skin flaps are dissected in a plane just external to the fascia of the underlying gluteal musculature. The superior flap is dissected to a point above the iliac crest, and the inferior flap is dissected below the infragluteal crease. Laterally, the iliotibial tract is exposed and incised.

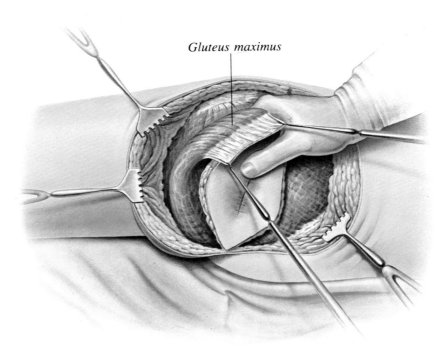

FIG. 5-34. The apronlike lateral insertion of the gluteus maximus muscle is next divided from its superior border down to and into the iliotibial tract. The divided gluteus maximus is then retracted medially to expose the underlying musculature, specifically the gluteus medius and piriformis muscles. Palpation of the gluteus maximus from the undersurface, as shown here, will allow the surgeon to determine the proper plane of dissection for the resection.

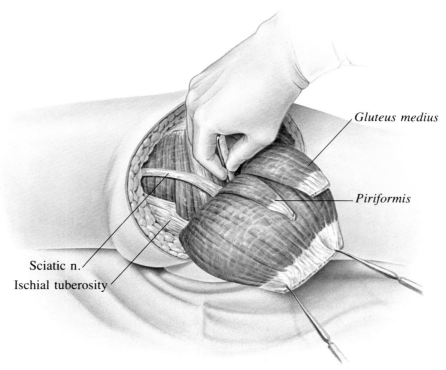

FIG. 5-35. The sciatic nerve is seen extending inferiorly from the lower border of the piriformis. When the plane anterior (deep) to the piriformis is selected, this muscle and a portion of the gluteus medius are divided laterally, and the plane anterior to this musculature is palpated. If it is determined that there is an inadequate margin at this plane, the procedure must be aborted and hemipelvectomy will then be performed (using the anterior skin flap shown on pp. 99 and 103). If the plane just described is clear, the limb-sparing buttock resection can be completed.

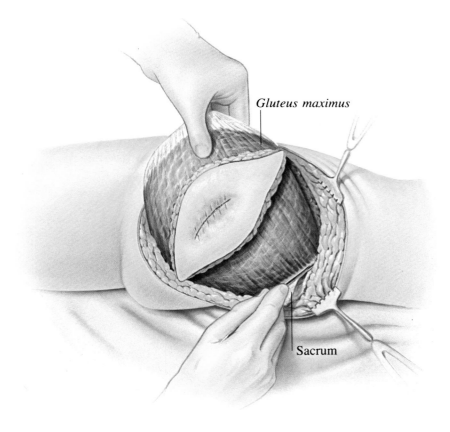

FIG. 5-36. If the margin anterior to the piriformis is determined to be adequate for the specific sarcoma, the origin of the gluteus maximus on the sacrum is next divided at the level of the bone, and the piriformis is divided at its insertion on the anterior surface of the distal sacrum.

95

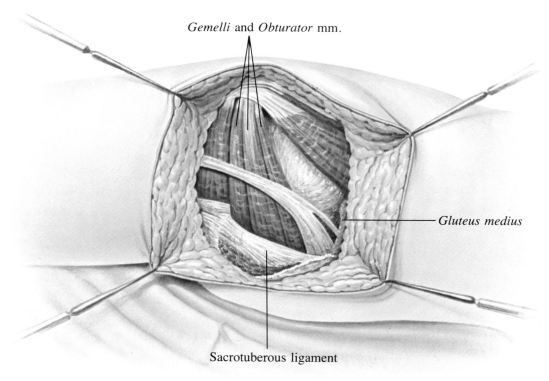

Gemelli and *Obturator* mm.

Gluteus medius

Sacrotuberous ligament

FIG. 5-37. The operative specimen has been removed exposing the obturator internus, the gemelli, and the remains of the gluteus medius behind the completely exposed sciatic nerve. The sacrotuberous ligament is also seen.

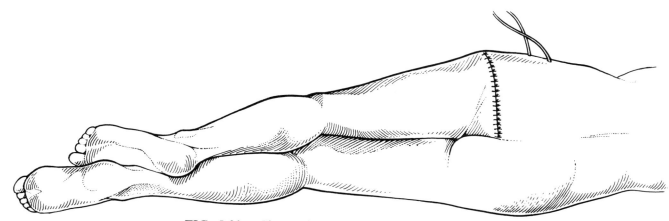

FIG. 5-38. Closure is accomplished after hemostasis is obtained and large suction catheters are inserted. If skin approximation is not possible, a rotation skin flap can be utilized with a split-thickness skin graft placed on the resulting defect.

Hemipelvectomy and Hip Joint Disarticulation

Girard (7) of Berne performed the first hemipelvectomy with survival of the patient in 1895, but Billroth had made a prior unsuccessful attempt to perform this operation in 1891. The terms employed to describe this operation have included *interinnominoabdominal amputation, hindquarter amputation,* and *disarticulation of the innominate bone,* but *hemipelvectomy* has achieved common usage over the years despite the fact it is a less accurate term than the others. The classic description of this procedure and its early history are included in the report of Gordon-Taylor and Wiles (8) in 1935. They described 5 patients for whom this procedure was employed as a single-stage operation and summarized the 79 amputations of this general type recorded in the literature. The operative mortality in their series was 2 out of 5 patients, while that following the 79 prior operations was 59.5%. George Pack reviewed his extensive experience with this procedure in 1956 (9), and his technique was well described in his book in 1958 (10). A later description of technique, with a summary of the world experience over more modern times, is that of Ravitch and Wilson (11) in 1964, who described 37 personal cases with 2 operative deaths. Since that time this operation, described by Gordon-Taylor as "one of the most colossal mutilations practiced on the human frame," has been employed infrequently, but with relative safety, for a number of clinical indications. These include malignant neoplasms of bone, soft-part sarcomas, selected patients with malignant melanomas, other cancers so situated anatomically that major amputation is required to achieve total resection, and a host of nonmalignant conditions including massive benign bone tumors, vascular malformations, radionecrosis of pelvic bones, trauma, and soft-tissue necrosis of infectious or vascular etiology.

For soft-part sarcomas, the specific indications for hemipelvectomy are purely anatomic ones. Sarcomas that arise in the proximal thigh, groin, or buttock are lesions that may be suitable for soft-part resection, rather than radical amputation, but the latter procedure may be required for these sites if a clear margin cannot be achieved by the lesser procedure. There are a number of modifications of the standard hemipelvectomy that relate to the specific location of the neoplasm and the structures involved. Large sarcomas and those lesions adjacent to or involving the femoral vessels or sciatic nerve frequently require radical amputation in order to achieve an adequate surgical margin around the neoplasm. An alternative amputation is disarticulation of the hip, but this is only applicable to lesions confined to the proximal thigh. Although this slightly less radical procedure may be technically feasible, it will usually provide a less adequate soft-tissue margin and involves transection of muscle and fascial planes already affected by the sarcoma just distal to the plane of dissection. Although the patient is able to sit more comfortably, and clothing may drape more naturally below the waist after hip joint disarticulation, hemipelvectomy or one of its modifications is preferable in most instances, owing to considerations relating to the margin achieved.

Modifications of the procedure of hemipelvectomy for sarcoma include the development of an anterior thigh skin flap for sarcomas of the buttock area requiring amputation (6) and the transection of the ilium and/or pubic rami rather than division of the sacroiliac joint and symphysis pubis (1,12). This latter procedure has some advantages for sarcomas in the proximal thigh that may not be adequately encompassed by hip joint disarticulation. Modifications of hemipelvectomy described for bone sarcomas arising in the pelvic bones include more limited local resection of the involved pelvic bone when feasible (4,5). Excision of the entire hemipelvis with preservation of the extremity has also been described for selected patients with bone lesions (3,13). Hemipelvectomy has been carried out in rare instances for other cancers involving pelvic wall structures, particularly recurrent cancer of the cervix, and the modification usually includes pelvic exenteration when this unusual operation is performed (2).

Rehabilitation of the patient following hemipelvectomy or hip joint disarticulation requires training in crutch walking early in the postoperative period. Often these patients feel more insecure at first than others requiring crutches, but the patient should be fully ambulatory on crutches by the time he or she is ready for hospital discharge. The other early rehabilitation required after hemipelvectomy is learning to sit comfortably, since the ischial tuberosity has been resected on the side of the amputation. This is facilitated with pillows or sponge-rubber pads fashioned for this purpose. The prosthesis employed for hemipelvectomy and hip joint disarticulation patients is cumbersome, and considerable training and practice are required to develop the skill needed to use it effectively for ambulation. This, plus initial tenderness of the operative area, leads us to discourage the fitting of a prosthesis until four to six months after operation. Some patients find the use of the prosthesis so awkward that they continue to use crutches for most activities. For elderly patients and patients with other physical limitations, it is often preferable to omit the prosthetic fitting and training.

References

1. Ariel IM, Shah JB: The conservative hemipelvectomy. Surg Gynecol Obstet 144:407–413, 1977.
2. Brunschwig A, Barber HRK: Pelvic exenteration combined with resection of segments of bony pelvis. Surgery 65:417–420, 1969.
3. Eilber FR, Grant TT, Sakai D, Morton DL: Internal hemipelvectomy—excision of the hemipelvis with limb preservation. Cancer 43:806–809, 1979.
4. Enneking WF, Spanier SS, Malawer MM: The effect of the anatomic setting on the results of surgical procedures for soft parts sarcoma of the thigh. Cancer 47:1005–1022, 1981.
5. Erickson U, Hielstedt A: Limb-saving radical resection of chondrosarcoma of the pelvis. J Bone Joint Surg 58-A:568–570, 1978.
6. Frey C, Matthews LS, Benjamin H, Fidler WJ: A new technique for hemipelvectomy. Surg Gynecol Obstet 143:753–756, 1976.
7. Girard Ch: Desarticulation de l'os iliaque pour Sarcome. Reve de Chir 15:952, 1895.
8. Gordon-Taylor G, Wiles P: Interinnominoabdominal (hindquarter) amputation. Br J Surg 22:671–695, 1935.
9. Pack GT: Major exarticulations for malignant neoplasms of the extremities: interscapulothoracic amputation, hip joint disarticulation, and interilioabdominal amputation. J Bone Joint Surg 38-A:249–262, 1956.
10. Pack GT, Ariel IM: Tumors of the Soft Somatic Tissues (A Clinical Treatise). New York, Paul B Hoeber, 1968, pp 105–122.
11. Ravitch MM, Wilson TC: Long-term results of hemipelvectomy. Ann Surg 159:667–682, 1964.
12. Sherman CD Jr, Duthie RB: Modified hemipelvectomy. Cancer 13:51–54, 1960.
13. Steel HH: Resection of the hemipelvis for malignant diseases. (An alternative to hindquarter amputation for periacetabular chondrosarcoma of the pelvis). Semin Oncol 8:222–228, 1981.

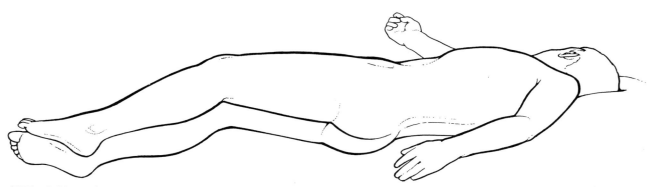

FIG. 5-39.   The patient is positioned with the affected limb slightly elevated by means of folded towels under the lumbar area; a Foley catheter is inserted into the bladder, and the anal opening is closed with a purse-string suture. In the male the scrotum is sutured to the opposite thigh, and the entire skin of the groin, buttock, perineum, and abdomen is prepared in the standard fashion. The lower extremity is prepped far enough onto the thigh to allow draping of the entire extremity so that it can be moved by the surgeon during the procedure.

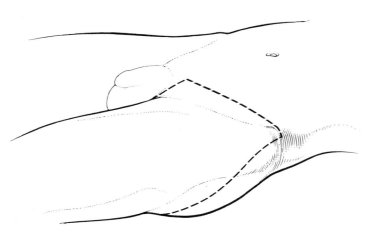

FIG. 5-40.   The anterior portion of the incision is made from a point just above the pubic tubercle extending upward and outward to a point just above the iliac crest. This incision is just above the inguinal ligament and is deepened to the external oblique fascia of the lower abdomen. Dissection of skin and subcutaneous fat inferiorly will expose the inguinal ligament in its entirety.

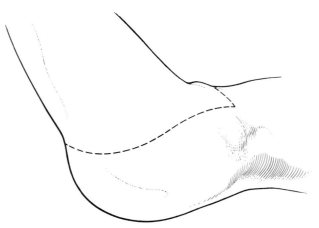

FIG. 5-41.   The posterior incision outlines a flap over the buttock and extends from the lateral extension of the anterior incision down into the infragluteal groove to the perineum. Here, it joins the anterior incision just lateral to the genitalia in the region of the symphysis pubis. Generally, this part of the incision is not made until the anterior dissection is complete and the surgeon is prepared to carry out dissection of the posterior skin flap over the gluteus maximus.

99

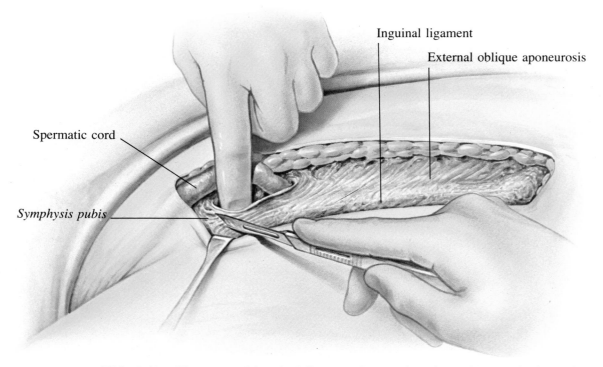

FIG. 5-42. The exposed inguinal ligament is detached from the symphysis pubis as shown here. The rectus abdominus is also divided at its insertion into the pubic bone. The peritoneum of the iliac area is exposed by this series of operative steps. Care should be taken to identify and preserve the spermatic cord in the male unless the extent of disease is an indication for its resection.

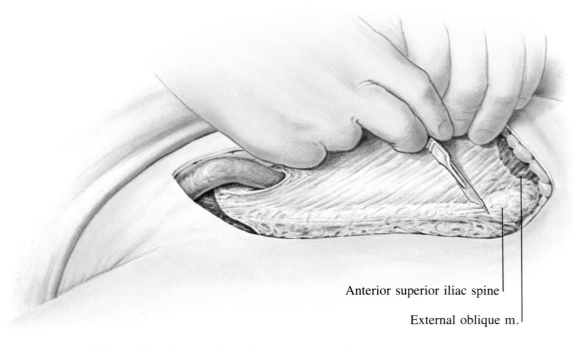

FIG. 5-43. The inguinal ligament is detached from the iliac crest at the anterior iliac spine. The abdominal wall musculature is then separated from the anterior part of the iliac crest.

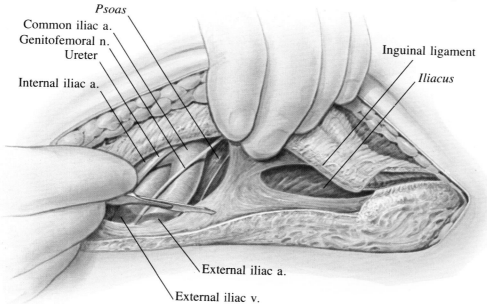

Psoas
Common iliac a.
Genitofemoral n.
Ureter
Internal iliac a.

Inguinal ligament
Iliacus

External iliac a.
External iliac v.

FIG. 5-44. The peritoneum is dissected medially to expose the iliac fossa and the ureter coursing over the iliac vessels at their bifurcation. The spermatic cord in males is preserved and retracted medially, as are the ureter and urinary bladder.

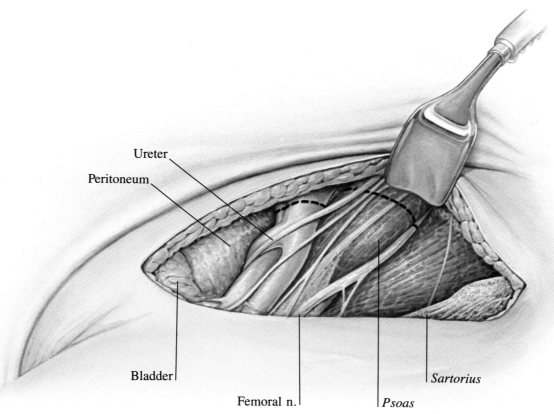

Ureter
Peritoneum

Bladder
Femoral n.
Psoas
Sartorius

FIG. 5-45. At this point in the procedure, an incision can be made in the peritoneum anteriorly to allow abdominal exploration to determine resectability and the absence of intraabdominal metastases. This peritoneal incision can then be closed if there are no findings that prevent the surgeon from proceeding with the hemipelvectomy. Generally, this step applies to melanoma more often than to sarcoma. The exposed common iliac artery and vein are individually isolated, ligated, suture-ligated, and divided. This site of the division may be distal to the bifurcation when appropriate, and then will include both external and internal iliac vessel ligations. Care is taken to avoid injury to the ureter. The psoas muscle and the femoral nerve are transected above this point at the level indicated. This will expose the underlying sacroiliac joint.

101

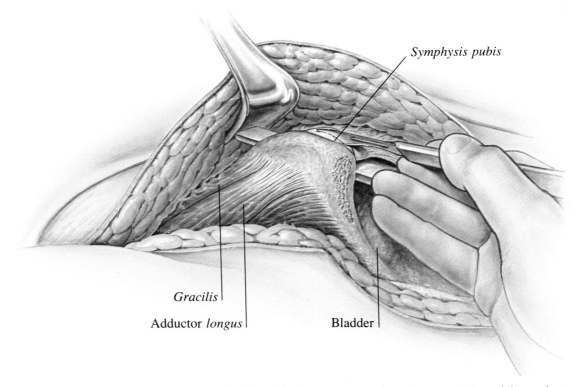

Symphysis pubis

Gracilis

Adductor *longus*

Bladder

FIG. 5-46. The symphysis pubis is now exposed, and a small tunnel is made on its posterior and inferior surface to allow division of this structure in the midline. This is accomplished with a scalpel in younger patients, owing to the cartilaginous nature of this structure, but a Gigli saw may be required in older patients. The tissues behind the symphysis, including the urethra and a venous plexus in this region, are protected with a malleable retractor during this division.

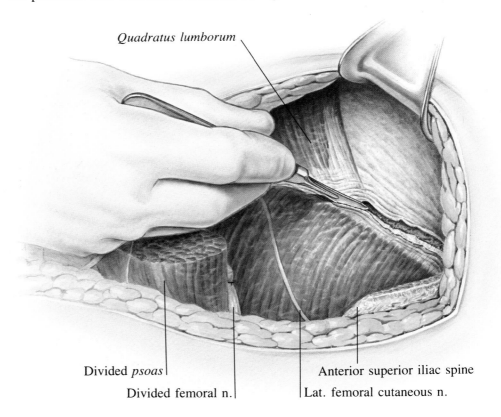

Quadratus lumborum

FIG. 5-47. The crest of the ilium is now skeletonized by severing the quadratus lumborum.

Divided *psoas*

Divided femoral n.

Anterior superior iliac spine

Lat. femoral cutaneous n.

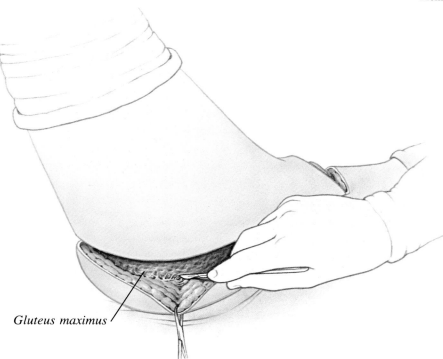

Gluteus maximus

FIG. 5-48. Before proceeding with sacroiliac disarticulation, the posterior flap is outlined as shown in Figure 5-41. A skin flap is dissected at the level of the fascia overlying the gluteus maximus as far posterior as the sacrum to allow the subsequent separation of this muscle from its origin on the sacrum. Exposure for this part of the operation is accomplished by medial rotation of the lower extremity, which has been draped "free" for this purpose.

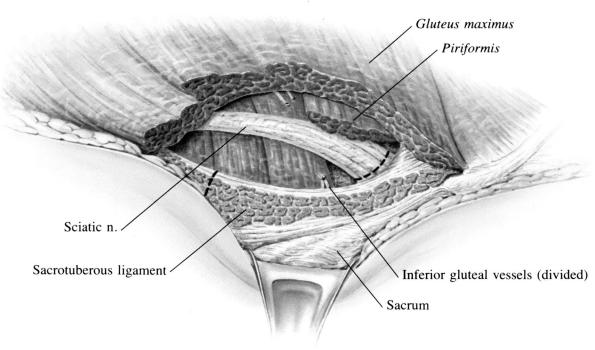

Gluteus maximus

Piriformis

Sciatic n.

Sacrotuberous ligament

Inferior gluteal vessels (divided)

Sacrum

FIG. 5-49. The origin of the gluteus maximus on the sacrum has been divided at the level of the bone, and the remaining major posterior structures divided now are the piriformis muscle, the sacrotuberous ligament, and the sciatic nerve. The superior and inferior gluteal vessels are secured during this part of the procedure. All that remains to be divided are the sacroiliac joint and the levator ani muscle sling.

103

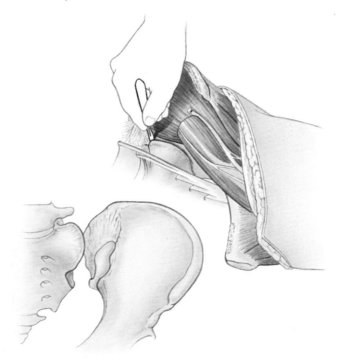

FIG. 5-50. The sacroiliac joint is divided with a scalpel or with the help of a chisel and leverage downward on the lateral aspect of the ilium to dislocate this joint. Care is taken at this point to avoid injury to the major intraabdominal structures. An appreciation of the obliquity of the sacroiliac joint is necessary to allow a proper line of division. In order to obtain a satisfactory margin in some cases, it may be necessary to transect the lateral portion of the sacrum itself.

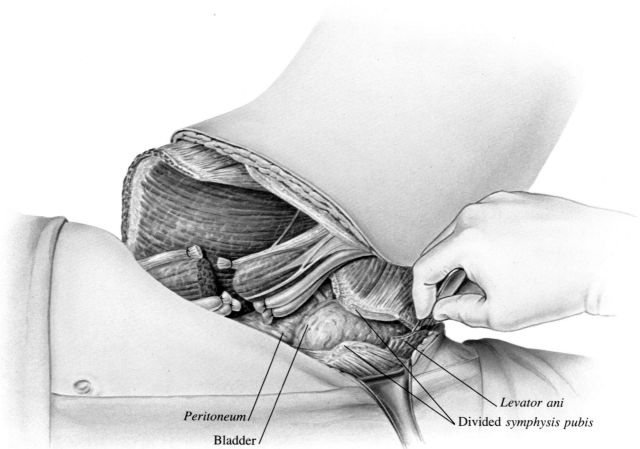

Peritoneum

Bladder

Levator ani

Divided *symphysis pubis*

FIG. 5-51. The remaining structure to be divided is the attachment of the levator ani muscles. The specimen is then removed. During this final portion of the operation, the extremity is rotated laterally and abducted.

104

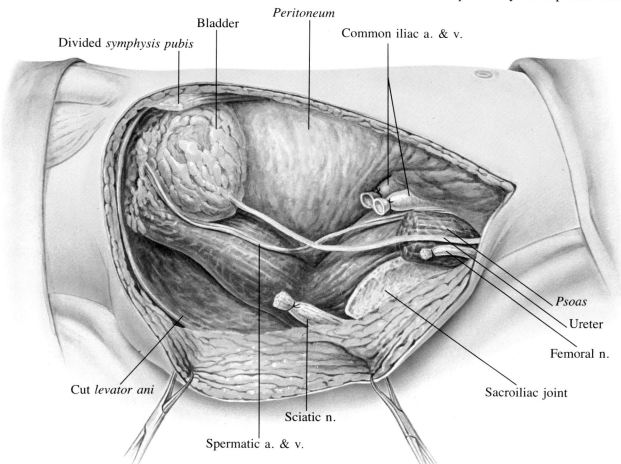

Divided *symphysis pubis* Bladder *Peritoneum* Common iliac a. & v.

Psoas

Ureter

Femoral n.

Sacroiliac joint

Cut *levator ani*

Sciatic n.

Spermatic a. & v.

FIG. 5-52. The operative field is exposed showing the sacral surface of the sacroiliac joint and the line of separation of the symphysis pubis. The peritoneum, bladder, and ureter are visualized as well as the ligated stumps of the iliac vessels.

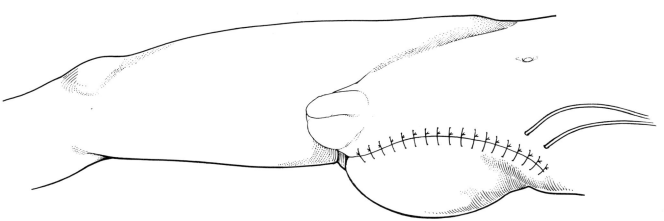

FIG. 5-53. After hemostasis has been obtained, closure is accomplished by uniting the large posterior flap to the abdominal skin and subcutaneous tissue anteriorly; the skin flaps serve as the only covering for the exposed peritoneum. Subcutaneous tissue closure is with interrupted sutures, and skin closure is with sutures or staples. Suction catheters are employed. If there is redundant tissue on the posterior flap, a V-shaped segment is removed. The suture used for temporary closure of the anus is removed at the end of the procedure.

105

Anterior Flap Variation for Hemipelvectomy

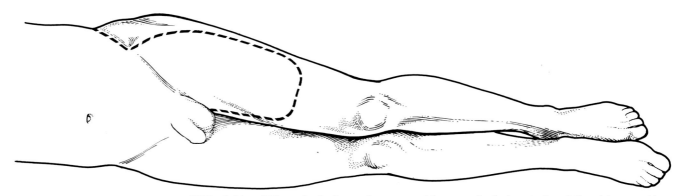

FIG. 5-54. When the lesion to be resected is posteriorly located and the skin resection required over the buttock is more extensive, an anterior skin flap may be used to allow closure rather than the standard buttock flap. This incision outlined on the anterior thigh preserves skin below the inguinal ligament and will require ligation of the femoral artery at a more distal point than described in the standard procedure. Ligation of the femoral vein also will be carried out more distally for the same purpose, that of preserving a blood supply to the anterior skin flap.

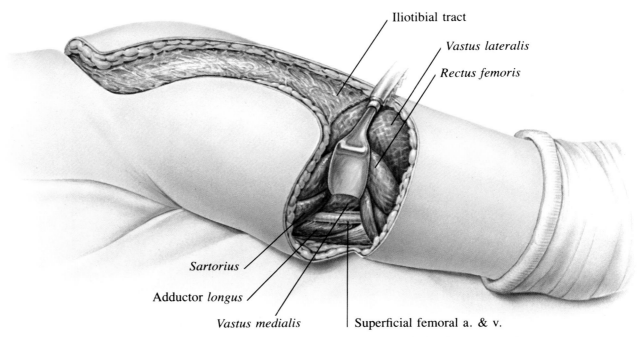

FIG. 5-55. The incision is carried through the fascia, and the sartorius is exposed in the midthigh. Retraction of the rectus femoris will expose the superficial femoral vessels as shown. A shorter anterior flap may be employed in some instances.

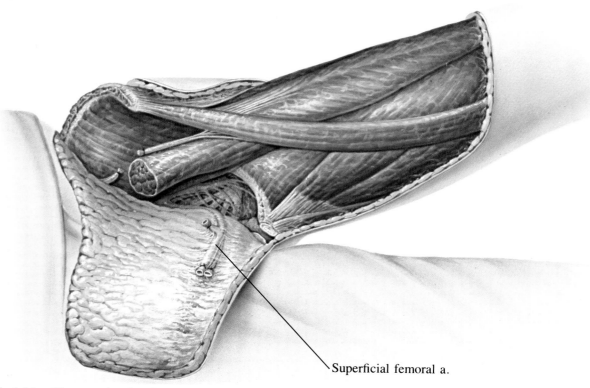

Superficial femoral a.

FIG. 5-56. The anterior flap is then mobilized with short segments of the preserved femoral vessels and their branches arising in the region of the femoral triangle. The procedure is carried out as described previously except for the resection of buttock skin and the preservation of the anterior thigh skin flap.

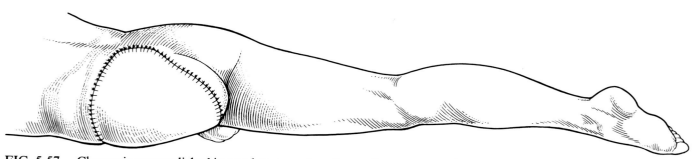

FIG. 5-57. Closure is accomplished in two layers, and suction catheters are employed for wound drainage.

Technique of Hip Joint Disarticulation

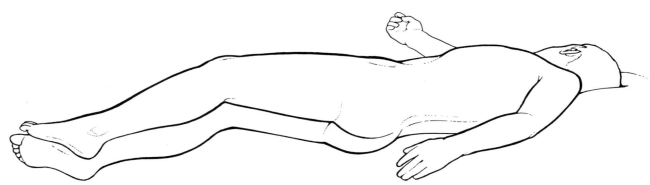

FIG. 5-58. This operation is rarely employed for soft-part sarcomas since a more adequate margin is usually obtained by hemipelvectomy for lesions that are not anatomically suited for soft-part resection. The patient is placed on the operating table, prepped, draped, and positioned in a manner similar to that shown for hemipelvectomy.

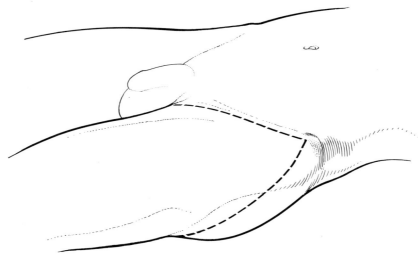

FIG. 5-59. The anterior incision is just below the inguinal ligament.

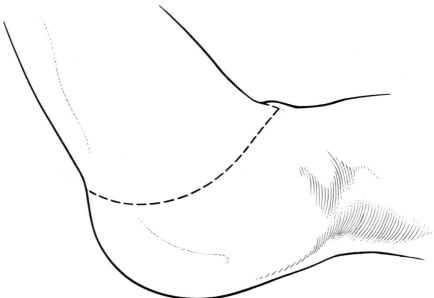

FIG. 5-60. The posterior incision is similar to that shown for hemipelvectomy, but it is placed slightly below the infragluteal crease.

108

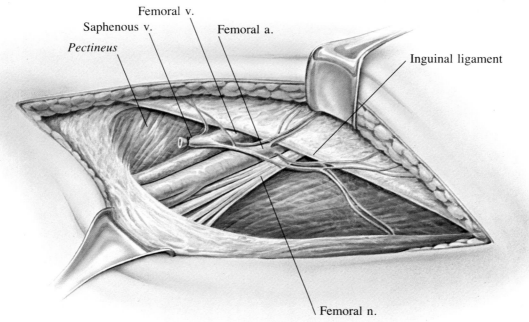

Femoral v.

Saphenous v.

Pectineus

Femoral a.

Inguinal ligament

Femoral n.

FIG. 5-61. The anterior incision is deepened through the subcutaneous tissues and fascia at the level of the inguinal ligament. Dissection of the two flaps created by the superior lateral extensions of the incision allows exposure of the lower abdominal wall, the inguinal ligament, and the vessels and nerve in the femoral triangle.

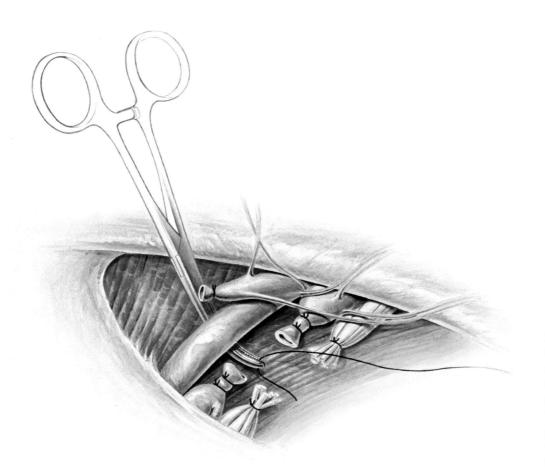

FIG. 5-62. The edge of the inguinal ligament is cleared, and the femoral artery and vein are dissected after opening the femoral sheath. These vessels are isolated, ligated, suture-ligated, and divided. The femoral nerve is transected at the same level.

109

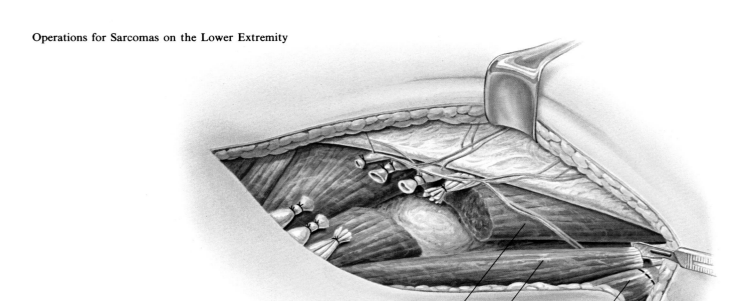

FIG. 5-63. The anterior thigh muscles are exposed at their origin from the iliac bone. The sartorius, quadriceps, and tensor fascia lata are divided at this point.

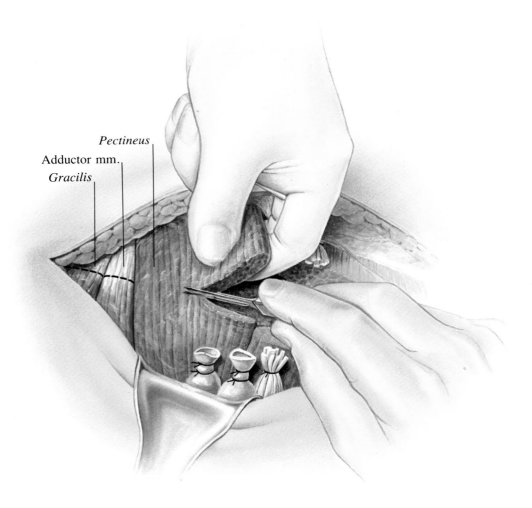

FIG. 5-64. The limb is now abducted and the medial muscles (gracilis, pectineus, and adductors) are transected.

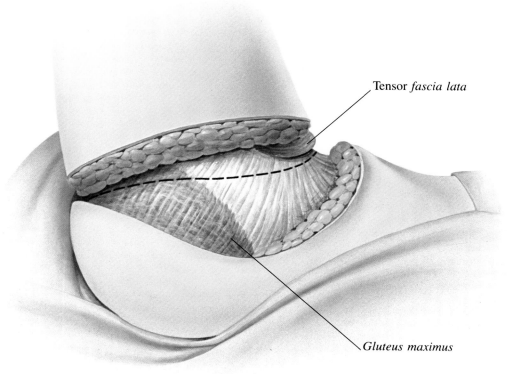

Tensor *fascia lata*

Gluteus maximus

FIG. 5-65.   The limb is now flexed and adducted to allow exposure of the posterior muscles requiring division. Transection of the gluteal muscles is accomplished at the level of the skin incision.

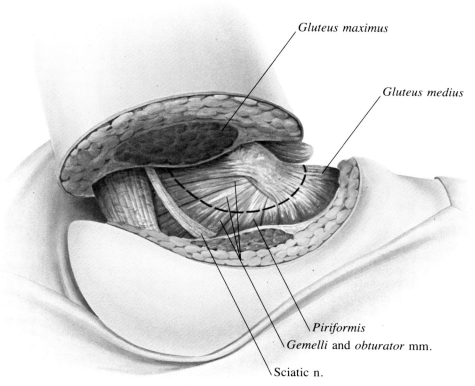

Gluteus maximus

Gluteus medius

Piriformis

Gemelli and *obturator* mm.

Sciatic n.

FIG. 5-66.   The muscles deep to the gluteus maximus (gluteus medius, piriformis, and gemelli) are transected prior to exposing the hip joint.

111

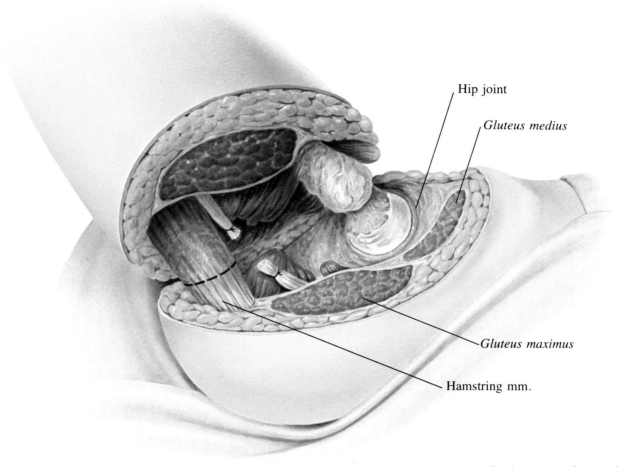

Hip joint

Gluteus medius

Gluteus maximus

Hamstring mm.

FIG. 5-67. The capsule of the hip joint is made taut by further adduction and internal rotation, and the capsule of the joint is then incised. The hamstring muscles and the sciatic nerve are transected next.

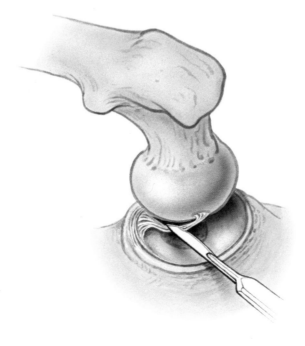

FIG. 5-68. The head of the femur is forced out of the acetabulum so that the round ligament can be divided.

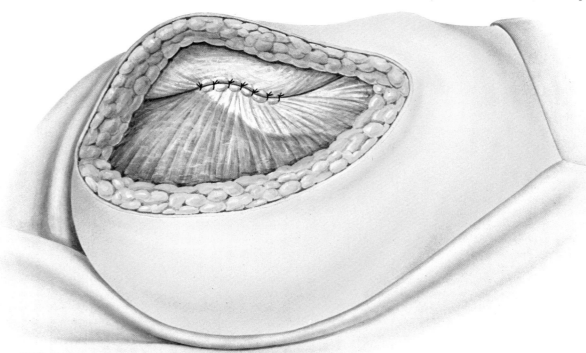

FIG. 5-69. Additional debridement of the muscular stumps is carried out and hemostasis obtained. The exposed acetabulum is covered by suturing adjacent muscles.

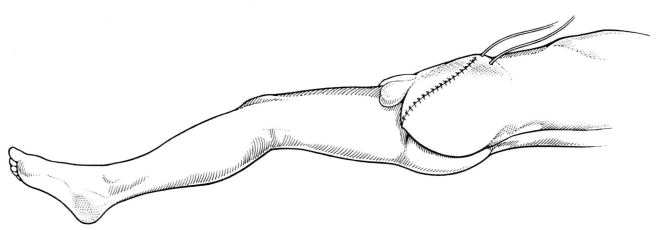

FIG. 5-70. Closure is accomplished with subcutaneous and skin sutures after placing suction catheters in the wound.

113

6 Operations for Sarcomas on the Chest and Abdominal Walls

Chest Wall Resection of Soft-Part Sarcomas

Soft-tissue sarcomas arising in the chest wall are unusual tumors which are difficult to manage owing to the limited thickness of the soft tissues overlying the ribs, rib cartilages, intercostal muscles, and sternum. Obtaining an adequate margin on these tissues often requires resection of the full thickness of the chest wall, and traditional repairs have included the use of fascia or prosthetic mesh to prevent functional disabilities (flail chest) (1–3,5–10). When a limited skin and chest wall resection has been performed, local skin flaps can be mobilized to obtain coverage over the chest wall closure. Recently, the use of myocutaneous flaps has provided more reliable replacement of extensive full-thickness chest wall defects (7). Flaps that can be used include the latissimus dorsi, pectoralis major, or rectus abdominis myocutaneous flaps (see Chapter 9). These flaps have the advantage of the use of autogenous, vascularized fascia to obtain a good chest wall closure, thus preventing paradoxical motion and potential late breakdown of the chest wall closure. In addition, adequate skin coverage is obtained. The resulting skin defect may be closed primarily or with a split-thickness skin graft. Another method of chest wall reconstruction includes the use of omentum (4). This can be rotated through the abdomen, thus not requiring a microvascular anastomosis, and can be placed on top of either fascia lata or synthetic mesh and covered with a split-thickness skin graft. These methods all enable the surgeon to perform a wide soft-part resection, thus decreasing the chance of local recurrence developing in these patients.

References

1. Boyd AW, Shaw WW, McCarthy JG: Immediate reconstruction of full-thickness chest wall defects. Ann Thorac Surg 32:337–346, 1981.
2. Dingman RO, Argenta LC: Reconstruction of the chest wall. Ann Thorac Surg 31:45–52, 1981.
3. Eschapasse H, Gaillard J, Henry F, Founiel G, Berthoumier F, Desrez X: Repair of large chest wall defects: experience with 23 patients. Ann Thorac Surg 32:329–336, 1981.
4. Jurkiewicz MJ, Arnold PG: The omentum: an account of its use in the reconstruction of the chest wall. Ann Surg 185:548–554, 1977.
5. Leonardi HK, Neptune WB: Surgical management of chest wall tumors. Am J Surg 139:569–574, 1980.
6. Lopez R, Didolkar MS, Karakousis C, Bakamjian V: Problems in resection of chest wall sarcomas. Am Surg 45:471–477, 1979.
7. McCormack P, Bains MS, Beattie EJ, Martini N: New trends in skeletal reconstruction after resection of chest wall tumors. Ann Thorac Surg 32:202–208, 1981.
8. Pradhan DJ, Musikabhumma S, Michelson E, Juanteguy JM, Wilder RJ: Total sternal resection and reconstruction using bone grafts and fascia lata. Am Surg 39:180–184, 1973.
9. Ramming KP, Holmes EC, Zarem HA, Lesavoy MA, Morton DL: Surgical management and reconstruction of extensive chest wall malignancies. Am J Surg 144:146–152, 1982.
10. Rees TM, Converse JM: Surgical reconstruction of defects of the thoracic wall. Surg Gynecol Obstet 121:1066–1072, 1965.

This patient has a sarcoma arising from the pectoralis major on the anterior chest wall. The proximity of the lesion to the underlying costal cartilages and associated intercostal muscles leads to a need for full-thickness resection of the chest wall to obtain an adequate margin.

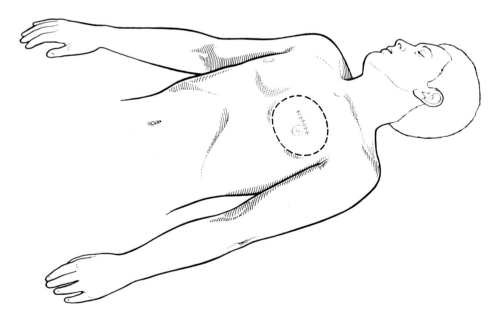

FIG. 6-1. The elliptical incision employed for this resection includes the skin and subcutaneous tissue around the previous incision that was utilized for excisional biopsy. An incisional biopsy would have been preferable to the enucleation that had been carried out, but the original surgeon thought this was a benign lipoma. The location of the incision employed and the margin will obviously vary with the individual case of sarcoma.

115

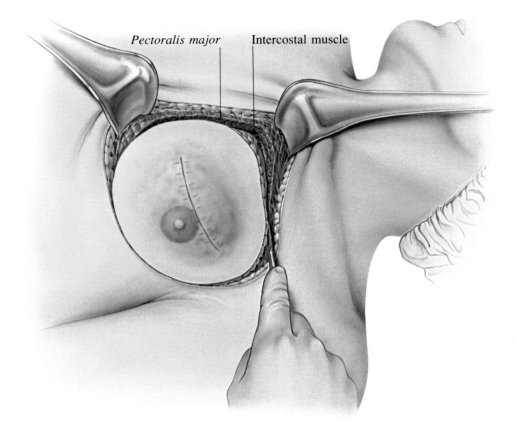

FIG. 6-2. The incision is carried down to the pectoralis major laterally, superiorly, and inferiorly, and down to the lateral edge of the sternum near the site of the origin of the pectoralis major.

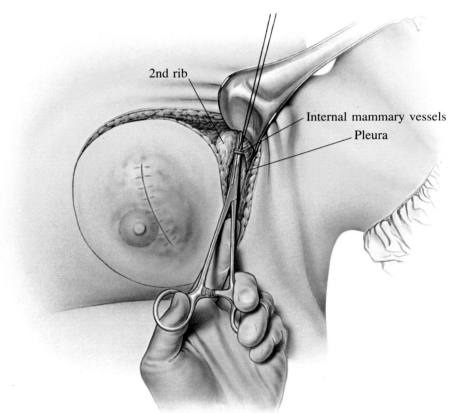

FIG. 6-3. The pectoralis major is divided over the second costal cartilage superiorly, since this is the superior margin of planned resection. In this case the second costal cartilage and a short segment of the adjacent rib are resected subperiosteally, and the internal mammary vessels are isolated for division.

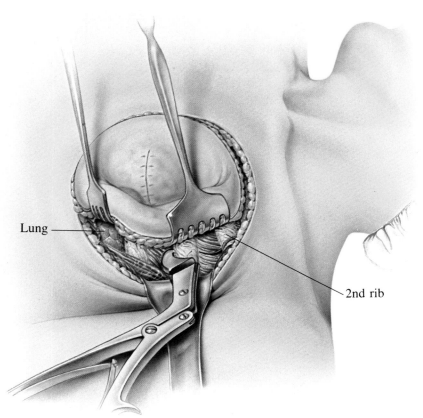

Lung

2nd rib

FIG. 6-4.   The fourth interspace is exposed and opened anteriorly in a similar fashion after transecting the overlying pectoralis major. The pectoralis major is next divided lateral to the proposed site of the chest wall resection. The third and fourth ribs are now approached laterally for transection (along with the adjacent intercostal muscles). Hemostasis is obtained by suture ligature of the intercostal vessel in each interspace.

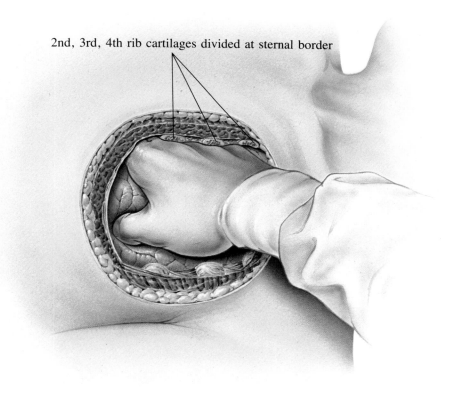

2nd, 3rd, 4th rib cartilages divided at sternal border

FIG. 6-5.   After ligation of the internal mammary vessels in the fourth interspace, the rib cartilages are divided at their attachment to the sternum using a scalpel. The surgical defect produced by this resection is shown with underlying lung tissue presenting. Inspection and palpation of the lung reveal no suspicious areas for metastasis.

117

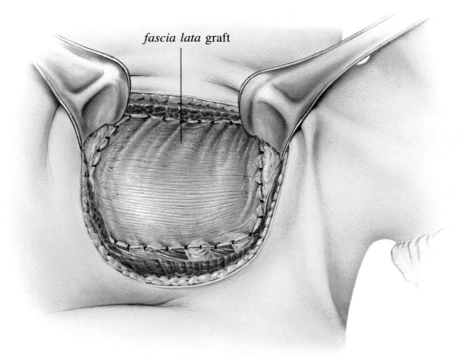

fascia lata graft

FIG. 6-6. Closure of the chest wall defect is accomplished by a large graft of fascia lata that was obtained from the lateral thigh. Initial fixation of the fascia to the sternum was accomplished with heavy sutures passed through the edge of the sternum; the lateral sutures are placed through intercostal muscle and around each of the transected ribs. Pressure on the lateral chest wall allows these sutures to be tied in such a way as to produce tension on the fascia lata and create a firm chest well closure. This is important to prevent paradoxical motion with respiration.

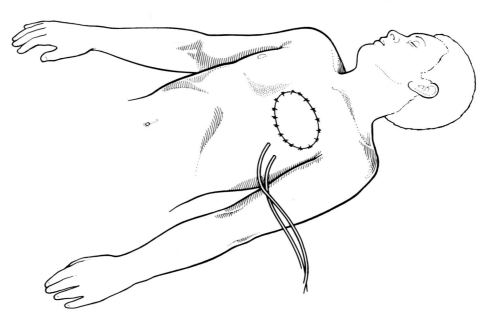

FIG. 6-7. Adequate skin is often made available for completing the skin and subcutaneous closure over the fascia lata by developing some form of bipedicle skin flap. A latissimus dorsi myocutaneous flap was employed in this instance, with a split-thickness skin graft applied to the resulting defect on the posterolateral portion of the chest wall. The myocutaneous flap shown here was tunneled under the skin laterally. The split-thickness graft is not visible due to its position (see Chapter 9 for details of this reconstruction).

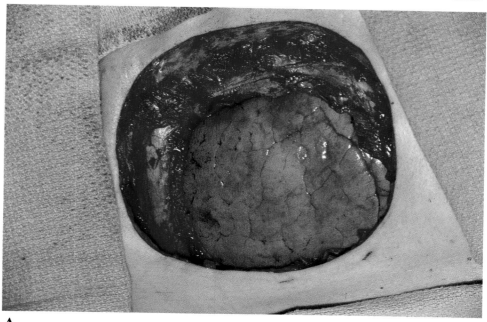

A

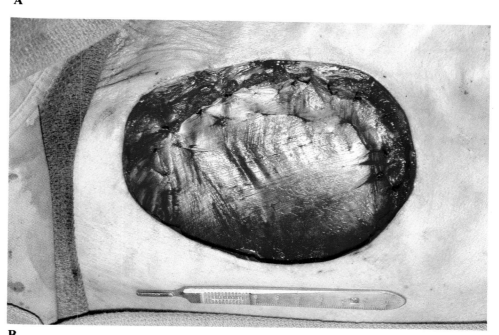

B

FIG. 6-8. Operative view after chest wall resection for a liposarcoma arising in the pectoral region of a 68-year-old male (**A**). This defect is similar to that in the operative procedure illustrated in Figures 6-1 to 6-7. The medial margin of resection seen superiorly is the sternal edge. The chest wall defect was closed with fascia lata graft (**B**), and skin closure was accomplished by a latissimus dorsi myocutaneous flap.

119

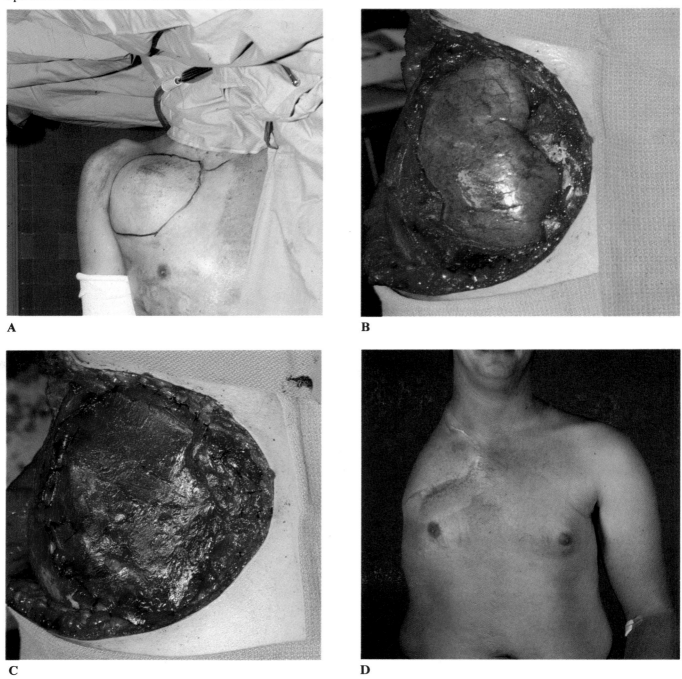

FIG. 6-9. Chest wall resection with interscapulothoracic (IST) amputation. This is a 22-year-old male with fibrosarcoma arising in the pectoral region. The plan for resection is IST due to local involvement of the neurovascular bundle in the axilla (**A**). Extension of the sarcoma to the chest wall required resection of the first three ribs in continuity with the soft-tissue resection. The resulting chest wall defect is shown at the completion of the procedure (**B**). A fascia lata graft was employed to close this chest wall defect (**C**). Primary closure was accomplished with the posterior skin flap (**D**). Postoperative irradiation was employed owing to the narrow (but clear) margin at the thoracic inlet.

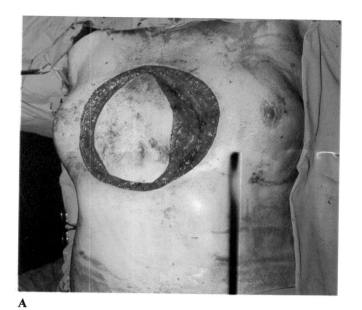

A

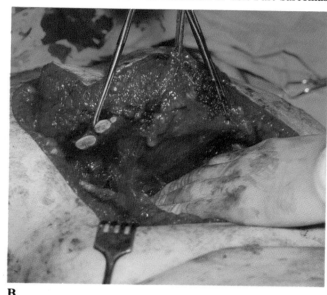

B

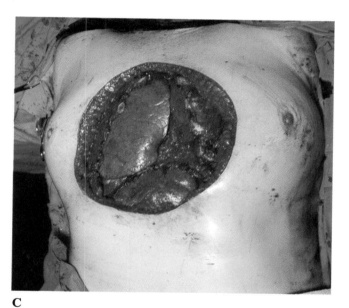

C

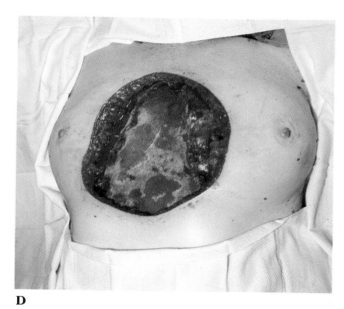

D

FIG. 6-10. Operative views of chest wall resection for a rhabdomyosarcoma arising in the sternum of a 55-year-old female. The soft-tissue resection was carried down to both pectoral muscles (**A**). The lesion did not extend through the sternum into the mediastinum, as seen at the time of transection of the costal cartilages of the right anterior chest wall (**B**). The entire sternal body and lower portion of the manubrium were resected, along with medial portions of the costal cartilages. The operative view of the completed dissection (**C**) demonstrates both lung and mediastinum. Synthetic mesh was used to close the chest wall defect (**D**), and final closure was accomplished in this case with local tissues (**E**).

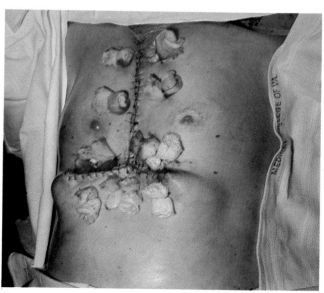

E

121

Abdominal Wall Resection
for Soft-Part Sarcoma

Sarcomas arising in the abdominal wall are unusual tumors which have been difficult to treat because of the problem of abdominal wall reconstruction. Abdominal wall tumors range from the relatively benign, slow-growing, non-metastasizing desmoid tumors (3) to the metastasizing sarcomas (3,4). The principles of wide soft-part resection, with removal of the entire fascial compartment surrounding the tumor, are much more difficult to obtain when managing abdominal wall tumors. Reconstruction has traditionally utilized prosthetic material or fascial autograft (1,2), with wide mobilization of the remaining abdominal wall as bipedicle flaps to obtain closure. Recently, we have used wide tensor fascia lata flaps (see Chapter 9) to reconstruct the entire abdominal wall. With this type of flap, no foreign tissue is required and total reconstruction is performed at the time of resection of the primary tumor. This has the advantage of reducing morbidity, obviating the need for further reconstructive procedures, reducing the length of hospitalization, and allowing earlier functional rehabilitation. In addition, the surgeon does not have to worry about whether or not the abdominal wall will be able to be reconstructed, thus ensuring wide resection of the primary tumor. Historical series of soft-part sarcomas arising in the abdominal wall have an overall recurrence rate of about 40% and a five-year survival rate of about 25%. Recurrence rates for desmoid tumors have been similar, thus further emphasizing the need for wide resection.

References

1. Karakousis CP: Exposure and reconstruction in the lower portion of the retroperitoneum and abdominal wall. Arch Surg 117:840–844, 1982.
2. McPeak CJ, Miller TR: Abdominal wall replacement. Surgery 47:944–952, 1960.
3. Pack GT, Ehrlich HE: Neoplasms of the anterior abdominal wall with special consideration of desmoid tumors. Int Abstr Surg 79:197–198, 1944.
4. Shiu MH, Flancbaum L, Hajdu SI, Fortner JG: Malignant soft-tissue tumors of the anterior abdominal wall. Arch Surg 115:152–155, 1980.

This patient had biopsy proof of a sarcoma involving the abdominal wall musculature. The operative plan was to resect a full-thickness segment of the abdominal wall with adequate margins around the sarcoma, since the preoperative CT scan seemed to indicate that the sarcoma was limited to the abdominal wall itself.

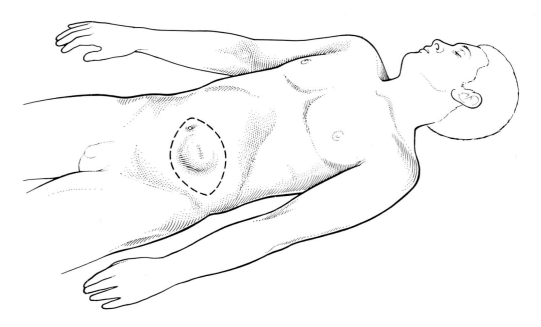

FIG. 6-11. The incision through the skin and subcutaneous tissue was made at an appropriate distance from the biopsy site.

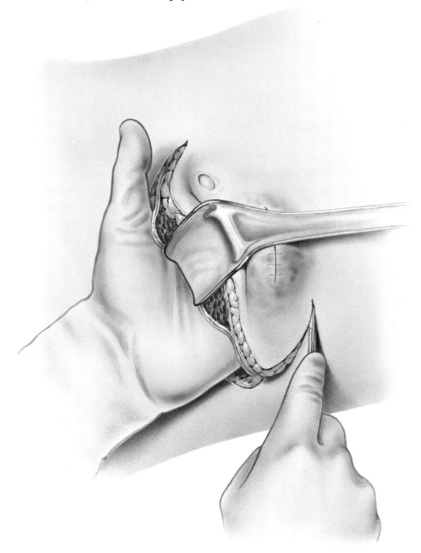

FIG. 6-12. The abdominal musculature and peritoneum are incised at one margin to allow exploratory laparotomy. This is to determine any penetration of the peritoneum by the sarcoma or the presence of intraabdominal metastases. Either would lead to modification of the procedure.

123

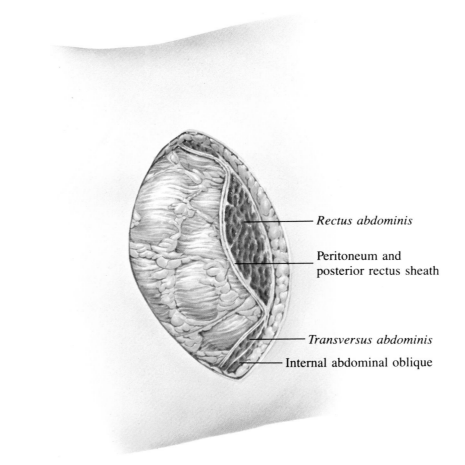

FIG. 6-13. Full-thickness excision of the abdominal wall, including skin, subcutaneous tissue, and musculature, with a corresponding disc of peritoneum, was then accomplished by sharp dissection. This is a view of the full-thickness surgical defect created in the abdominal wall.

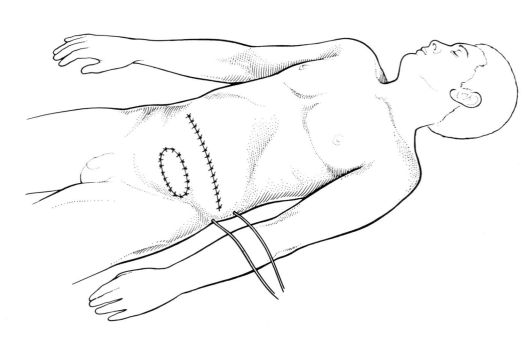

FIG. 6-14. In this instance Marlex mesh was utilized to replace the abdominal wall musculature. Undermining the subcutaneous tissue and developing a bipedicle flap was necessary to obtain skin closure over the Marlex mesh. A split-thickness skin graft was performed to cover the resulting skin defect produced by movement of the bipedicle flap. A useful alternative method of closure for many abdominal wall defects is the tensor fascia lata myocutaneous flap (see Chapter 9).

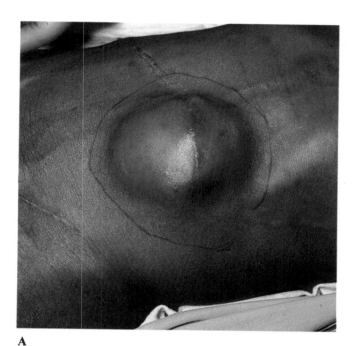
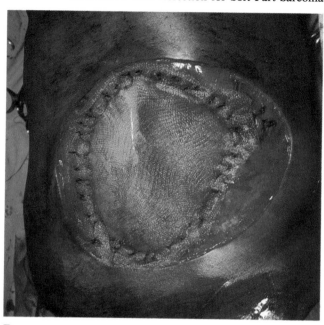

A
B

FIG. 6-15. Malignant neurilemmoma arising from the abdominal wall in a 50-year-old male patient with von Recklinghausen's neurofibromatosis (**A**). The full-thickness defect created by abdominal wall resection was closed with a synthetic mesh prosthesis prior to skin closure (**B**).

125

7 Retroperitoneal Sarcomas

Soft-tissue sarcomas arising from the retroperitoneum are rare, comprising 10%–20% of all cases in most series of soft-tissue sarcomas in adults. (Retroperitoneal sarcomas in children are discussed in Chapter 13). When considering malignant tumors of the retroperitoneal space, other than those arising in the kidney or adrenal gland, the incidence of soft-tissue sarcomas ranges from 43% to 70%, with lymphomas comprising from 15% to 32% of the total (4,7). Much less common malignant tumors of the retroperitoneal area, such as malignant paragangliomas and malignant teratomas, account for the remainder. Retroperitoneal soft-tissue sarcomas represent both a diagnostic and therapeutic dilemma because of their silent growth, the large size they reach before they are detected, and their poor prognosis despite aggressive therapy.

The most frequent histologic varieties of retroperitoneal sarcoma in adults are liposarcoma and leiomyosarcoma, with fibrosarcoma or malignant fibrous histiocytoma being next in incidence (1,9). Earlier reports do not include malignant fibrous histiocytoma, since the disease was first described only in recent years. Less common retroperitoneal sarcomas include rhabdomyosarcoma, lymphangiosarcoma, malignant schwannoma, and hemangioendothelioma. These tumors tend to present as an asymptomatic abdominal mass found during routine physical examination or, more frequently, as an abdominal mass associated with vague abdominal complaints that reflect the displacement or partial compression of some portion of the gastrointestinal or genitourinary tract. Sarcomas arising in the pelvic portion of the retroperitoneum often produce symptoms due to pressure on the bladder, rectum, or sacral nerve plexus. Weight loss, gastrointestinal obstruction, and unilateral or bilateral leg edema are frequently observed in most advanced cases. Whether symptomatic or not, a palpable abdominal mass is the most frequent physical finding in patients with retroperitoneal sarcomas; pelvic and rectal examination may corroborate pelvic involvement if it is present.

Diagnostic work-up of patients suspected of having a malignant retroperitoneal neoplasm generally focuses on anatomic studies of the extent of the mass and the involvement of adjacent structures in the retroperitoneum or abdomen. In the past, radiologic contrast studies of the upper and lower gastrointestinal tract and visceral angiography usually were employed to reveal displacement of normal anatomy and to detect abnormal patterns of vascularization in the region of the sarcoma. These studies were generally incomplete, from the standpoint of providing useful information on the actual extent of the tumor, and newer imaging techniques have proven to be much more useful. Ultrasonography and computed tomography of the abdomen and pelvis are now the most rewarding diagnostic studies for the initial evaluation of the patient when a retroperitoneal tumor is suspected.

Noninvasive radiologic studies using ultrasonography and computed tomography usually show a large single or multilobulated mass that is primarily solid but frequently contains some cystic components. We have found computed tomography to accurately delineate size, extent of tumor, and contiguity to adjacent structures as well as being useful in assessing displacement or obstruction of kidney or ureter by the sarcoma (8). The relationship of the lesion to major blood vessels also can be assessed by these imaging techniques, and they have proven to be the most accurate radiologic procedures for planning the operative approach for patients with retroperitoneal sarcomas. Diagnostic needle biopsy of the retroperitoneal lesion can be accomplished in conjunction with these imaging methods. However, we believe this percutaneous approach to diagnosis should be limited to patients not deemed to be candidates for major surgery on the basis of radiologic or clinical findings.

Treatment of retroperitoneal sarcoma is primarily operative, since neither radiotherapy nor chemotherapy is capable of offering a possibility of long-term control of the lesion. All patients with potentially resectable retroperitoneal sarcomas should undergo exploratory laparotomy, since a transperitoneal approach is the most likely route for achieving complete resection. Although the anatomic location of the sarcoma and the structures involved may preclude complete resection of the lesion, all reported series demonstrate that unresected disease is uniformly fatal. Thus, the operative plan should be that of complete resection of the sarcoma and the adjacent structures involved by the lesion, if this is technically possible.

The appropriate surgical procedures are frequently complex because the sarcoma tends to involve several intraabdominal structures and usually will require an "en bloc" resection of the sarcoma along with the organs that are invaded or attached to the lesion (segments of the large and small intestines, pancreas, kidney, or spleen). In selected cases the inferior vena cava (6), pelvic organs (partial or total pelvic exenteration), or segments of the abdominal or pelvic walls (hemipelvectomy) must be resected in order to completely remove the neoplasm.

In spite of the magnitude of the surgical procedure that is often required, the basic concept of "wide local excision with a margin of normal tissue" that has been so well established in the management of sarcomas of the extremities can seldom be applied as well to retroperitoneal sarcomas. The proximity of important structures (superior mesenteric vessels, aorta, spine, etc.) often tends to limit the margin of resection and is undoubtedly the reason for high rates of local treatment failure. In reported series, complete excision of the tumor has been achieved in half to two-thirds of the patients who appear to have potentially resectable lesions on preoperative evaluation (1–5). Nevertheless, local recurrence does develop in a large proportion of patients in whom "total" resection is accomplished.

Radiation therapy and chemotherapy following incomplete surgical excision do not appear to change the generally poor outlook for retroperitoneal sarcomas. The role of these modalities as potential adjuvant therapy following grossly complete excision of the tumor has not yet been established. The relative infrequency of retroperitoneal sarcomas, the limited tolerance of the normal tissues in the abdomen (stomach, liver, kidney, and bowel) to "curative" doses of radiotherapy, and the ineffectiveness of currently available drug regimens for large soft-tissue sarcomas in adults have discouraged meaningful studies of such combined-therapy regimens. Despite the potential palliative benefit of these nonoperative measures, resection remains the primary treatment for this group of neoplasms.

Despite the generally poor prognosis for retroperitoneal soft-tissue sarcomas, long-term control is achieved in some instances. As with sarcomas arising in other sites, the overall disease-free survival rates depend on both the histologic grade of the sarcoma and the completeness of the excision. In patients with low-grade sarcomas (particularly liposarcoma) reexcision of recurrent tumor can often be repeated several times over a period of years, resulting in relatively long-term survival despite ultimate treatment failure. From the standpoint of histologic type, liposarcomas seem to have the best prognosis, particularly the low-grade ones, but the overall probability of cure with these lesions is much lower than that observed with similar tumors arising in the extremities (20% disease-free survival at five years and 12% at ten years for retroperitoneal primaries). Leiomyosarcomas and malignant fibrous histiocytomas are associated with a uniformly poor prognosis, with almost no survivors at the five-year interval. In those patients failing treatment, distant metastasis is found in approximately half, but death from retroperitoneal sarcomas is usually the result of extensive intraabdominal disease leading to gastrointestinal bleeding, obstruction, perforation, and obstructive uropathy rather than problems associated with the metastasis.

References

1. Abbas JS, Holyoke ED, Moorer R, Karakousis CP: The surgical treatment and outcome of soft tissue sarcoma. Arch Surg 116:765–769, 1981.
2. Bengmark S, Hafstron L, Jonsson P, et al: Retroperitoneal sarcoma treated by surgery. J Surg Oncol 14:307–314, 1980.
3. Binder SC, Katz B, Sheridan MFB: Retroperitoneal liposarcoma. Ann Surg 187:257–261, 1978.
4. Cody HS III, Turnbull AD, Fortner JG, Hajdu SI: The continuing challenge of retroperitoneal sarcomas. Cancer 47:2147–2152, 1981.
5. Kinne DW, Chu FCH, Huvos AG, Yagoda A, Fortner JG: Treatment of primary and recurrent retroperitoneal liposarcoma: 25 year experience at Memorial Hospital. Cancer 31:53–64, 1973.
6. McPeak CJ: Resection of inferior vena cava and graft replacement (aortic homograft) for retroperitoneal sarcoma. Surgery 50:778–781, 1961.
7. Moore SV, Aldrete JS: Primary retroperitoneal sarcomas: the role of surgical treatment. Am J Surg 142:358–361, 1981.
8. Neifeld JP, Walsh JW, Lawrence W Jr: Computed tomography in the management of soft tissue tumors. Surg Gynecol Obstet 155:535–540, 1982.
9. Storm FK, Eilber FR, Mirra J, Morton DL: Retroperitoneal sarcomas: a reappraisal of treatment. J Surg Oncol 17:1–7, 1981.

Retroperitoneal Sarcoma Arising in the Left Upper Quadrant

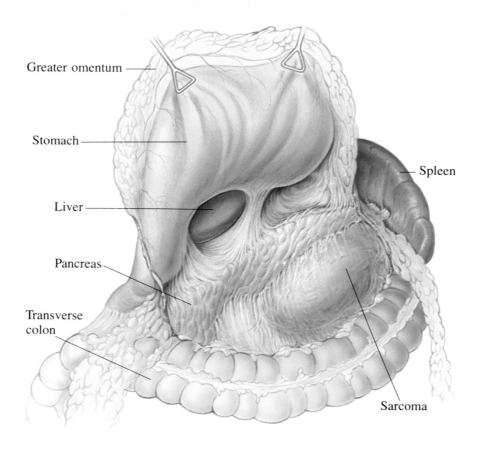

Greater omentum

Stomach

Liver

Pancreas

Transverse colon

Spleen

Sarcoma

FIG. 7-1. This retroperitoneal sarcoma appears to arise from the left retroperitoneal space behind the body and tail of the pancreas. After making a generous midline incision and carrying out abdominal exploration, the greater omentum is dissected from the transverse colon. The vasa brevia are divided, the stomach is retracted superiorly, and the lesser sac is well exposed. The retroperitoneal sarcoma has displaced the body and tail of the pancreas anteriorly, and it appears to involve the spleen and the adjacent mesocolon.

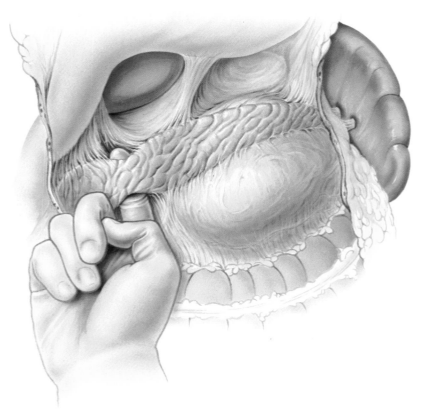

FIG. 7-2. Since the spleen and distal pancreas are adherent to the underlying neoplasm laterally, the pancreas and splenic vessels will require division. An incision is made inferior to the pancreas just lateral to its neck and the superior mesenteric vessels; a tunnel behind the body of the pancreas and splenic vessels is developed by gentle blunt dissection.

129

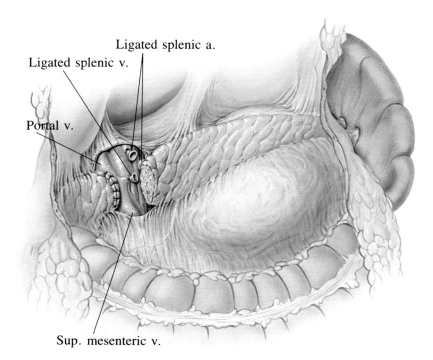

FIG. 7-3. The splenic artery and vein are isolated, divided, ligated, and suture-ligated. The pancreas is next transected, obtaining hemostasis with multiple through-and-through silk sutures that are tied across the cut surface of the pancreas. An attempt is made to identify and ligate the transected pancreatic duct, but this may be difficult and is not mandatory.

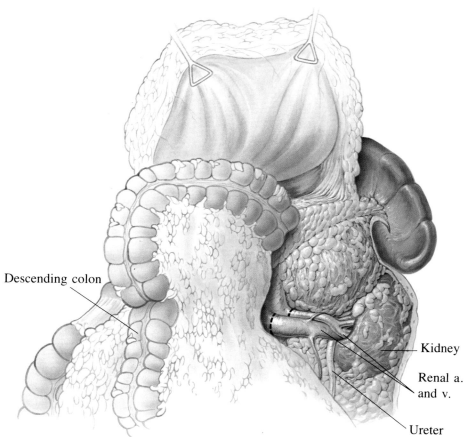

FIG. 7-4. The ligament of Treitz is next divided and the duodenum is retracted medially. Although a segment of mesocolon is attached to the underlying sarcoma, the vascular arcade of the left colon can be preserved in this patient. The splenic flexure and left colon are reflected medially. Palpation of the retroperitoneum demonstrates the sarcoma free of the aorta, but it is intimately adherent to the left kidney. Dissection proceeds superiorly to expose the renal vessels, which are isolated, divided, and individually ligated. All major vasculature to the tissues to be resected has now been controlled.

130

Diaphragm

Spleen

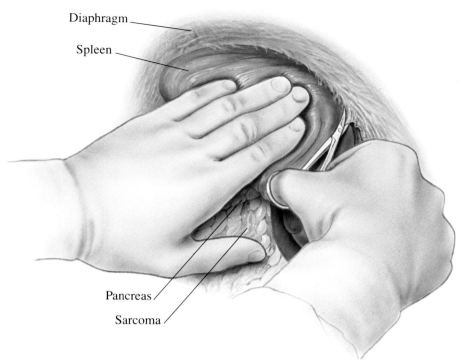

Pancreas

Sarcoma

FIG. 7-5. Mobilization of the specimen is now achieved by incision of the lateral peritoneal attachments of the spleen and downward and medial mobilization of the spleen, tail of pancreas, and lateral aspect of tumor mass.

Splenic a. & v.

Renal a. & v.

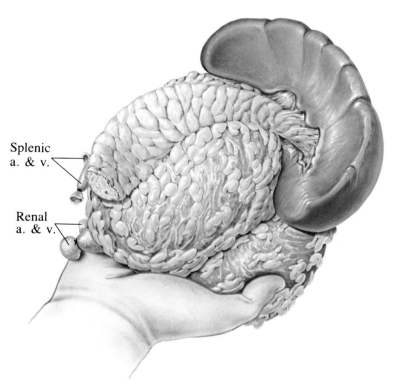

FIG. 7-6. The retroperitoneal plane behind the sarcoma and the kidney is next dissected by blunt dissection, freeing the spleen, kidney, adrenal, body and tail of the pancreas, and the neoplasm from the retroperitoneum and diaphragm. Smaller blood vessels (including the testicular/ovarian vessels) are divided and the specimen is removed.

131

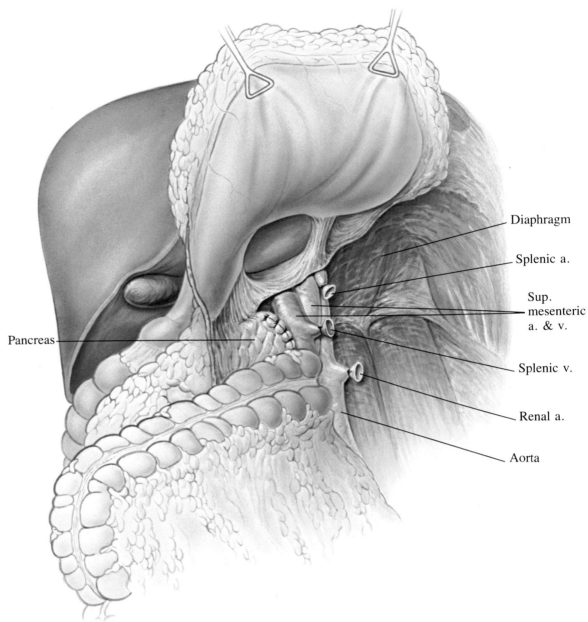

Diaphragm

Splenic a.

Sup.
mesenteric
a. & v.

Pancreas

Splenic v.

Renal a.

Aorta

FIG. 7-7.   The operative field after removal of the specimen. The diaphragm, retro-peritoneal musculature, and aorta are clearly seen.

132

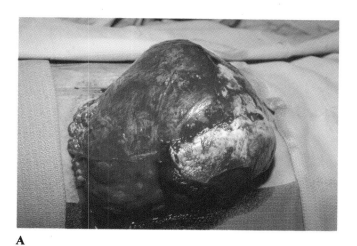

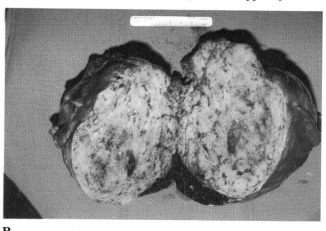

A

B

FIG. 7-8. Massive leiomyosarcoma of the retroperitoneal space at the time of operative exposure of the lesion (A). The spleen and the body and tail of the pancreas were resected with the sarcoma. The spleen is seen at the lower portion of the bisected surgical specimen (B).

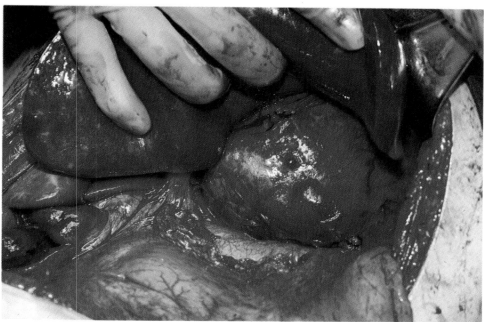

FIG. 7-9. Operative view of a retroperitoneal leiomyosarcoma arising from the paraaortic and retrohepatic area in a 20-year-old female. Anatomic location precluded adequate surgical margins, a frequent operative problem with retroperitoneal sarcomas.

133

Sarcoma Arising in the Right Retroperitoneal Space

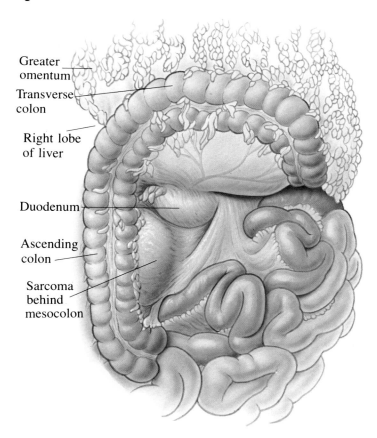

Greater omentum
Transverse colon
Right lobe of liver
Duodenum
Ascending colon
Sarcoma behind mesocolon

FIG. 7-10. A long midline incision is made, as preoperative work-up has outlined a large right retroperitoneal mass extending inferiorly from the level of the right kidney. This sarcoma does arise from the right retroperitoneal space and is palpable through the adjacent mesocolon. The ascending colon, hepatic flexure, duodenum, and right lobe of the liver are all displaced anteriorly by the mass. Careful abdominal exploration has failed to reveal metastases to the liver, peritoneum, or other sites.

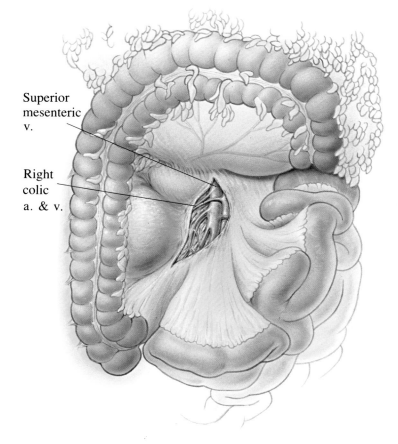

Superior mesenteric v.
Right colic a. & v.

FIG. 7-11. Since the key feature in the determination of resectability of the sarcoma is the relationship of the neoplasm to the superior mesenteric vessels and the vena cava, this area is evaluated by incising the mesocolon medial to the ileocolic vessels in a manner similar to that employed for right hemicolectomy. This incision is extended superiorly to the superior mesenteric vessels and duodenum, and digital exploration posteriorly and superiorly appears to demonstrate that the neoplasm is not attached to the underlying vena cava.

134

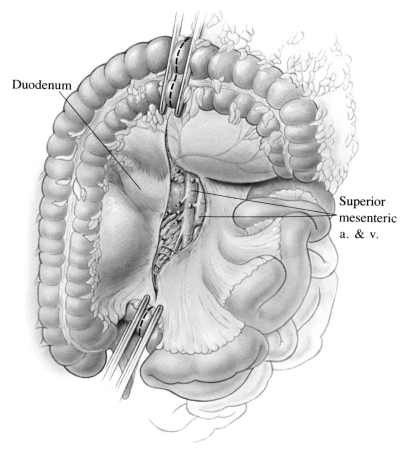

Duodenum

Superior
mesenteric
a. & v.

FIG. 7-12. Since it is planned to proceed with resection, the ileocolic and right colic vessels are ligated and divided adjacent to the superior mesenteric vessels. The transverse mesocolon is divided lateral to the right branch of the middle colic artery after the omentum is dissected superiorly off the transverse colon. The distal ileum and right side of the transverse colon are next clamped and divided, since resection will then include the blood supply of this portion of the colon.

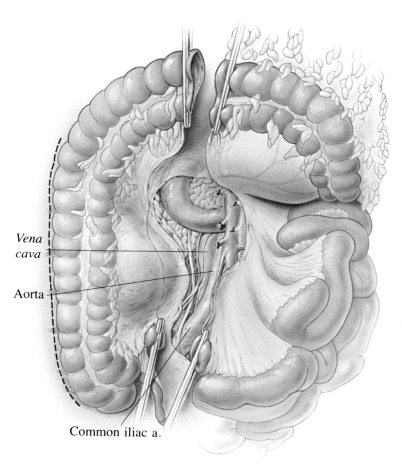

Vena
cava

Aorta

Common iliac a.

FIG. 7-13. The small bowel mesentery is retracted to the left side of the abdomen exposing the third portion of the duodenum, the inferior vena cava, aorta, and right common iliac vessels. When such a tumor extends across the midline it is bluntly dissected from these vessels by developing a plane adjacent to the adventitia. Superiorly the renal vessels are seen.

135

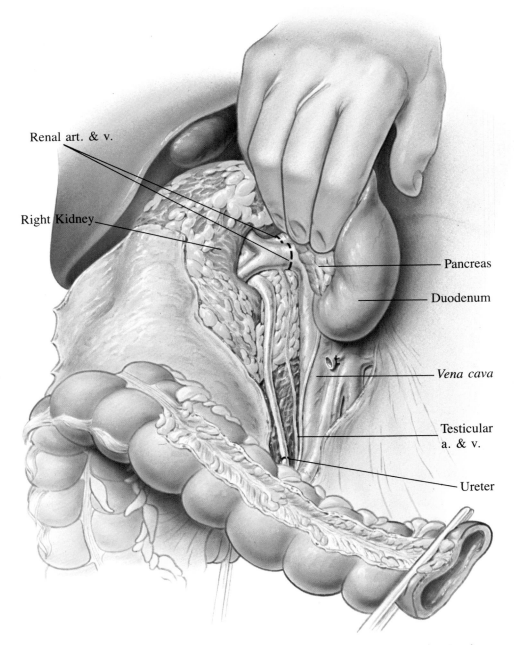

Renal art. & v.

Right Kidney

Pancreas

Duodenum

Vena cava

Testicular a. & v.

Ureter

FIG. 7-14.   The hepatic flexure of the colon is mobilized, exposing the duodenum and pancreas, which are retracted medially. The parietal peritoneum is incised lateral to the colon from the subhepatic region to the cecum. Since the sarcoma is juxtaposed to the lower pole of the kidney, it is resected en bloc with the sarcoma. This view shows mobilization of the right colon, the sarcoma, and the kidney while the pancreas and duodenum are displaced medially.

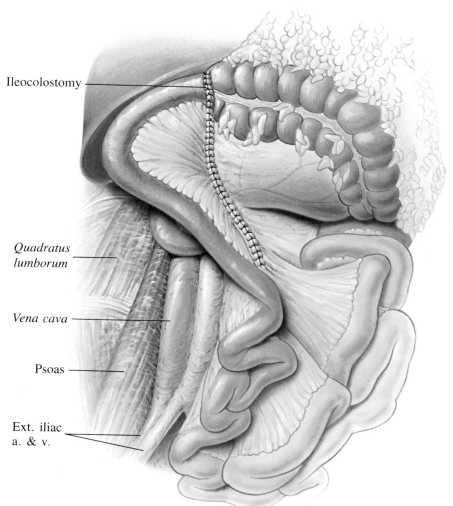

Ileocolostomy

Quadratus lumborum

Vena cava

Psoas

Ext. iliac
a. & v.

FIG. 7-15. By sharp and blunt dissection the tumor mass, en bloc with the kidney and right colon, is dissected from the lumbar and iliac fossa. If the psoas muscle is adherent, it is also removed. The ureter and spermatic/ovarian vessels are divided in the pelvis. In this diagram the field of dissection is seen after removal of the operative specimen. An ileocolostomy is next performed, the mesenteric window is repaired, and the abdomen closed without drains. The lumbar vessels, the posterior aspect of the psoas, inferior vena cava, right iliac vessels, and distal ligated ureter are all shown as well as the adjacent duodenum and pancreas.

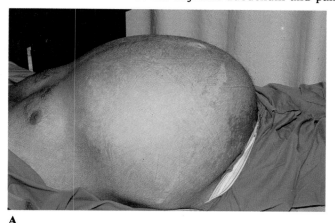

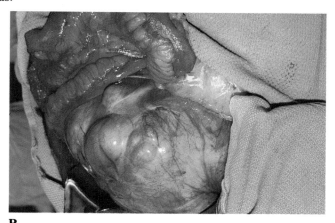

A

B

FIG. 7-16. Abdominal distension due to recurrent retroperitoneal liposarcoma in a 55-year-old male (**A**). The operative view shows the displacement of the colon by this large neoplasm (**B**).

137

Sarcoma Involving the Small Bowel Mesentery

FIG. 7-17. After the sarcoma involving the mesentery is noted, the abdominal cavity is carefully explored for the presence of metastases. The key to resectability of a lesion in this location is the relationship of the neoplasm to the superior mesenteric artery and vein. Exposure of the sarcoma is first accomplished by lifting the greater omentum, transverse colon, and mesocolon ventrally and superiorly. The peritoneum of the small bowel mesentery is incised adjacent to the superior mesenteric vessels to determine the presence or absence of involvement of these structures by the neoplasm. This sarcoma involves several branches of the superior mesenteric artery and vein, but the major trunks are "free." The tumor is mobile and unattached to the underlying retroperitoneal structures.

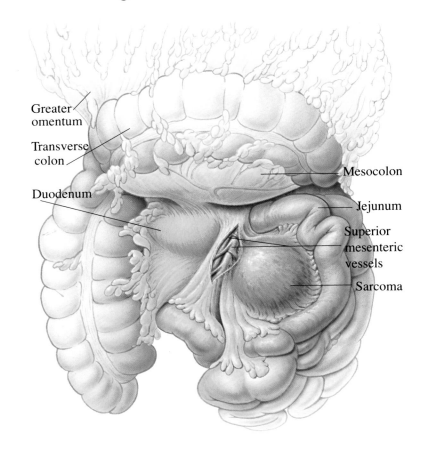

FIG. 7-18. The proximal branches of the superior mesenteric artery and vein which supply the segment of involved mesentery are ligated individually at their origins and divided. A portion of jejunum will require resection because of this devascularization.

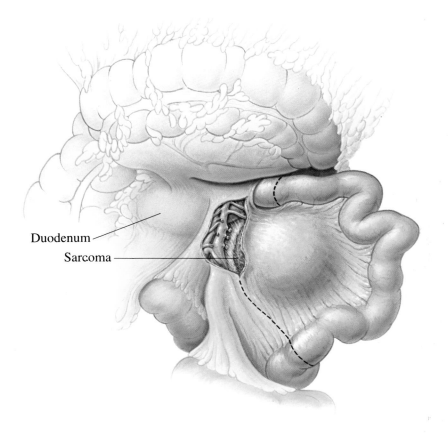

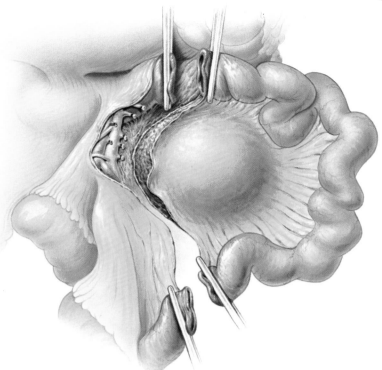

FIG. 7-19.   The duodenum is divided just to the left of the superior mesenteric vessels, and the mesentery is incised distal to the sarcoma and the divided intestinal branches. This mesenteric incision is carried out to the distal jejunum at a point that is assured an intact blood supply. The jejunum is divided.

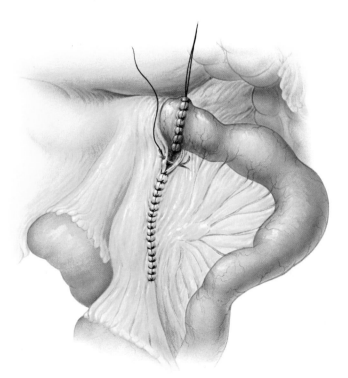

FIG. 7-20.   The mesentery containing the tumor and the associated jejunum has been removed. The distal jejunum is anastomosed to the duodenum and the mesenteric window closed.

139

8 Soft-Tissue Neoplasms of the Head and Neck

The vast majority of head and neck cancers are epithelial in origin, with primary mucosal squamous cell carcinomas the most common. Thyroid cancer, salivary gland cancer, and the lymphoreticular diseases are less frequent forms of cancer, while malignant neoplasms of mesodermal origin are relatively rare. These lesions are more frequent in children than in adults.

All the histologic types of benign and malignant soft-part neoplasms described in Chapter 1 occur in the head and neck, as in other sites, but they are less frequent in this anatomic area. The "fibromatoses" observed range from a histologically benign-appearing lesion, or variant of fasciitis, to fibrosarcoma (Fig. 8-1). The latter may present as a well-differentiated lesion on histologic examination and only manifest local recurrence after inadequate excision, or as the more undifferentiated fibrosarcoma or malignant fibrous histiocytoma capable of distant metastasis. Rhabdomyosarcoma occurs rarely in the head and neck region in adults, but this site accounts for roughly one-third of such lesions in childhood (see Chapter 13). Benign vascular lesions (hemangiomas and hygromas) are quite common in children, while angiosarcomas (Kaposi's sarcoma, malignant hemangioendothelioma, and malignant hemangiopericytoma) are occasionally found in the head and neck region in adults. Of the neural neoplasms, various benign forms of neurofibroma or neurilemmoma are relatively frequent in the head and neck region (Fig. 8-2), particularly in patients with the hereditary disorder von Recklinghausen's disease. However, malignant tumors arising from peripheral nerves are infrequent. Any of the less common soft-part sarcomas occurring elsewhere in the body (synovial sarcoma, liposarcoma, leiomyosarcoma, mesenchymoma, alveolar soft-part sarcoma, etc.) may arise anywhere in the head and neck region, but all are rare entities (7,20).

For all of the aforementioned lesions, the same principles of treatment apply for the head and neck as are employed in other anatomic regions of the body, but obvious physical and cosmetic limitations produce management restrictions, particularly those relating to wide resection (Fig. 8-3). In the soft tissues of the neck, it may be possible to obtain adequate margins by procedures similar to those generally employed for neck dissection, but sarcomas arising in the region of the mandible, maxilla, and base of the skull may prove challenging to the surgeon. Many of the innovative methods developed for reconstruction of surgical defects in the head and neck after operations

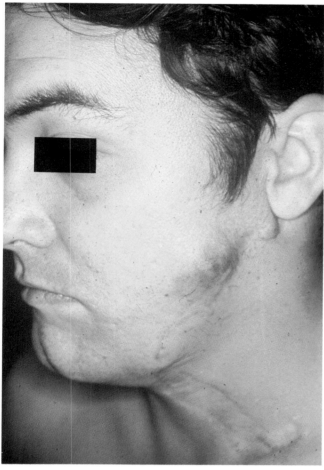

FIG. 8-1.   Low-grade fibrosarcoma of cheek in a 25-year-old male requiring mandibular resection for local control.

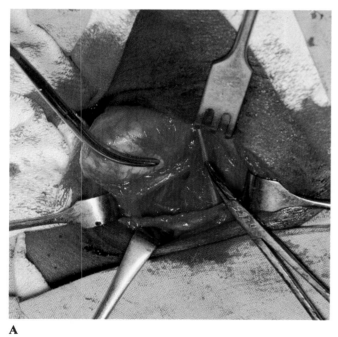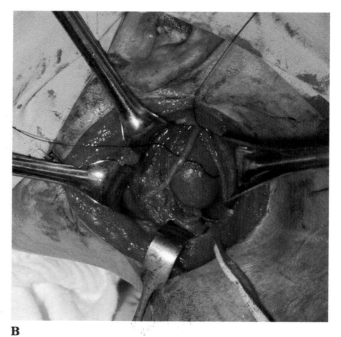

A   **B**

FIG. 8-2.   Malignant neurilemmoma (low grade) arising from region of the brachial plexus **(A)** and a grossly similar benign one from the cervical region **(B).**

141

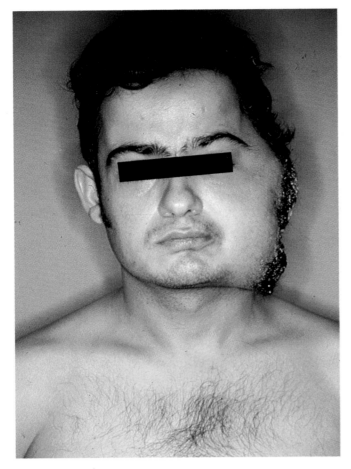

A

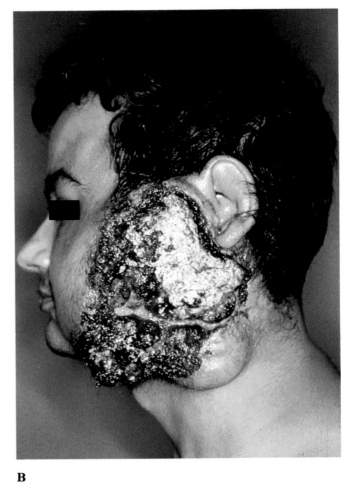

B

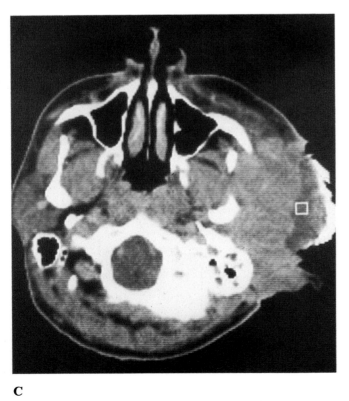

C

FIG. 8-3. Massive soft-part sarcoma in a 30-year-old male (**A** and **B**), with CT scan showing extent of disease (**C**). Radiation therapy produced complete regression of this lesion.

for carcinoma are particularly relevant to operations for soft-tissue sarcomas. These reconstructive operations are briefly described in Chapter 9, but the reader is referred also to texts on these approaches when they are applied for the much more common epithelial lesions arising in the head and neck area (1,10,15).

In addition to the variety of soft-tissue sarcomas that are described in Chapter 1, various neuroectodermal tumors, paragangliomas, and juvenile angiofibromas occur as uncommon soft-tissue neoplasms that are unique to the head and neck region. These lesions often create special problems in management and will be described in more detail.

Neuroectodermal Tumors

This group of neoplasms includes neuroblastoma, esthesioneuroblastoma, meningioma, and invasive retinoblastoma. The term *neuroblastoma* is an umbrella term covering a spectrum of histologic types of neurogenic neoplasms which take their origin from cells derived from the embryonic sympathetic neuroblasts, neural crest remnants, and the mantle layer of the neural tube. Thus, they may originate in the adrenal gland or in the sympathetic ganglia of the cervical, posterior mediastinal, retroperitoneal, or pelvic region. Neuroblastomas also arise from the cervical region in children, but such a lesion in the neck is more often a manifestation of metastasis from an extracervical primary site than a primary neoplasm.

Esthesioneuroblastoma is a neurogenic tumor of the olfactory region that arises in the roof of the nasal cavity (12). These rare tumors have been described in all age groups, with an equal incidence for both sexes. The tumor usually presents as a polypoid nasal mass, or masses, producing nasal obstruction, epistaxis, and anosmia. The true diagnosis is usually totally unsuspected clinically, and the lesion is initially treated as a benign polyp in most instances.

Meningiomas constitute 14% of all intracranial tumors, but extracranial and extraspinal meningiomas unassociated with neuraxial lesions are rare. The most frequent primary sites for meningioma in the head and neck are in the bones of the skull, the scalp, the orbit, the nose, the paranasal sinuses, and the middle ear.

Retinoblastomas also belong to this family of primitive neuroectodermal tumors; their incidence is relatively high in infants.

Excisional treatment is appropriate for most of these neurogenic tumors, but esthesioneuroblastoma deserves special comment. Both radical maxilloethmoidectomy and radiation therapy have been utilized as treatment for these lesions. However, when used alone, neither modality has resulted in permanent control of the disease in most patients. The combined use of radiation and surgery has produced a disease-free survival rate at five years of 33%, and treatment failures have local recurrence as the common denominator (2). The involvement of the cribriform plate and the extension of disease into the anterior cranial fossa is not adequately managed by the standard operative approach, since this is a common site of failure. A combined intracranial-extracranial approach might provide a greater likelihood of local control, but has not been the approach used in most retrospective series reported.

Paragangliomas of the Head and Neck

The extraadrenal paraganglia, derived from neural crest cells, make up an extensive and multicentric organ system. Neoplasms arising from nonchromaffin tissue in the neck (chemodectomas) are certainly uncommon, and less

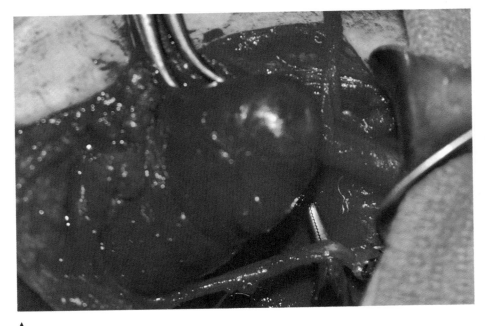

A

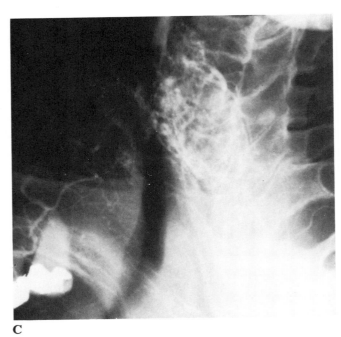

B

C

FIG. 8-4. Carotid body tumor demonstrated at the time of operation. The common carotid artery and vagus nerve are seen (**A**). The carotid angiogram demonstrates separation of the external and internal carotid arteries (**B**) and the increased vascularity (**C**) that is a classic finding with this lesion.

than 5% of these lesions ever develop malignant change in most series, despite higher reports in a few. Histologic appearance is not useful for determining malignant change, but size and rate of growth may be a clue. Both lymphatic and hematogenous metastases have been reported (6). These tumors arise from the region of the carotid body (13,19) at the bifurcation of the carotid artery (Fig. 8-4), the cervical portion of the vagus nerve (ganglion nodosum) (16) (Fig. 8-5), the jugular bulb (glomus jugulare), and the middle ear (11,21). The carotid body is the dominant site.

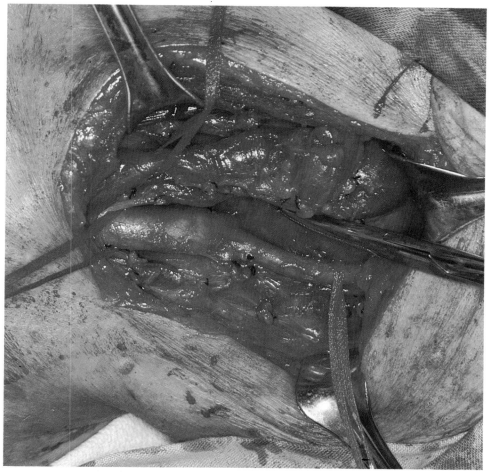

FIG. 8-5. Chemodectoma arising from the vagus nerve seen at the time of operation.

The overwhelming majority of chemodectomas that occur in the neck present either as an asymptomatic pulsatile mass near the angle of the mandible or as a cervical mass that bulges into the pharynx. Cranial nerve deficits may be present with larger lesions. Although the anatomic location of the neoplasm is essentially the same whether the lesion originates from the vagus nerve or the carotid body, it is of interest that the lesions originating from the vagus nerve often bulge into the pharynx, whereas those originating from the carotid body are usually felt more easily on external palpation. A bruit may be present also. Chemodectomas rarely produce increased levels of catecholamines, and hypertension is rarely observed with this group of neoplasms.

The differential diagnosis of cervical chemodectoma includes other possible causes of a neck mass, as well as carotid artery aneurysm. A characteristic of these tumors is their vascularity, and needle biopsy should be avoided when this diagnosis is suspected. Carotid angiography demonstrates a characteristic radiographic picture in chemodectomas that can establish this diagnosis with confidence (Fig. 8-4). The blood supply characteristically is from the external carotid artery.

In view of the generally benign nature of chemodectomas, the rarity of metastases, and the frequent absence of symptoms other than the physical presence of a mass, one must consider the treatment plan with great care. Dissection of a carotid body lesion from the carotid artery itself may be

145

difficult, but dissection in the subadventitial plane will usually allow resection without requiring vascular reconstruction. Ligation of the external carotid artery, the major source of blood supply, may be required to accomplish resection of larger lesions (13). Resection of a chemodectoma originating from the vagus nerve usually produces a greater nerve deficit than was present preoperatively, since it is virtually impossible to separate the tumor from the nerve. For these reasons, our general policy has been to carry out a surgical resection of chemodectomas only in young and middle-aged patients, and to studiously avoid a surgical approach in asymptomatic patients who are elderly. If there is progressive enlargement of the mass or some additional symptoms produced by the physical presence of the mass, surgery should be considered for the older patient as well.

About 10% of patients with chemodectomas develop synchronous or metachronous contralateral primary tumors; therefore, these patients should be kept under periodic observation. Bilaterality is more frequent with familial cases. This same neoplasm originating from the glomus jugulare is even more uncommon than the lesions just discussed. It usually causes symptoms relating to secondary middle ear involvement (tinnitus, vertigo, or bleeding from the external ear). The surgical approach for these lesions is similar to that for radical mastoidectomy.

Nasopharyngeal Angiofibromas

Juvenile angiofibromas are uncommon, nonmetastasizing neoplasms of mesodermal origin that are highly vascular, noninfiltrating, and arise in the nasopharynx and posterior nasal cavity. They are seen almost exclusively in adolescent males, and seldom are found in patients over 25 years of age. The marked predilection of this tumor for the adolescent male has always raised the suspicion of a possible endocrine abnormality in its causation. Detailed endocrine studies and urinary assays for ketosteroids and other metabolites have failed to demonstrate abnormal findings in this group of patients (9). Recently,

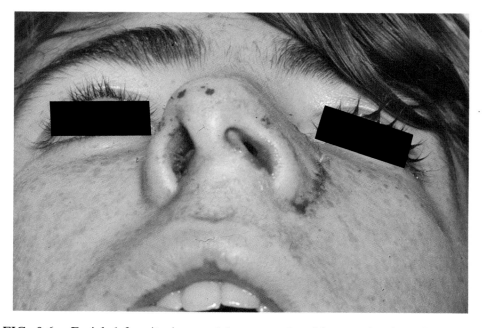

FIG. 8-6. Facial deformity in an adolescent male with extensive juvenile angiofibroma.

146

androgen binding activity ("receptor") has been shown to be present in some tumors (14), but the significance of this finding remains to be determined.

This tumor usually arises from the boundaries of the sphenopalatine space as a submucosal mass. As the tumor enlarges in the submucosa, it fills the posterior nasal cavity and flattens the turbinates posteriorly; it then extends into the nasopharynx and becomes visible behind the soft palate. The continuous growth of this neoplasm will destroy the pterygoid plate by pressure, and it then extends into the pterygomaxillary space. From there, the tumor may extend into the cheek anteriorly, thus producing the facial deformity that is seen in some patients (Fig. 8-6). The infratemporal region and the middle cranial fossa become involved eventually, leading to major problems in management (3,17).

A young male patient with repeated episodes of epistaxis and a nasopharyngeal mass must be assumed to have a nasopharyngeal angiofibroma. Nasal obstruction, rhinorrhea, and hypacusia may develop during the course of the disease. Biopsy of the mass will establish the diagnosis, but due to the possible severity of hemorrhage, it is recommended that biopsy be performed in the operating room after the appropriate preliminary radiographic studies. A coronal polytomogram will help in delineating the extent of the tumor and the degree of bone involvement. Carotid angiography with subtraction films will provide important information regarding the blood supply. Of great importance is the fact that these tumors have a classic angiographic pattern (Fig. 8-7) which may establish the pretreatment diagnosis without the hazard of biopsy (4,17).

Angiofibromas often can be resected completely by a skillful surgeon or may be treated with radiation as a temporizing measure. They may regress completely after the patient reaches 20 years of age.

Surgical resection can be accomplished with complete removal of the tumor in most cases. A transpalatine approach provides good exposure if the tumor is small or if the major component is within the nasal cavity.

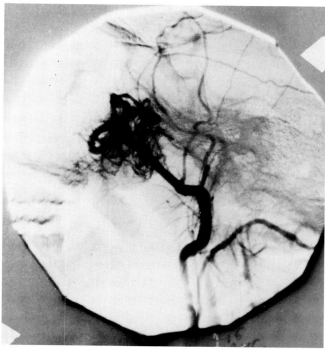

FIG. 8-7. Angiogram of juvenile angiofibroma.

For larger neoplasms with significant extension into the maxillary antrum or the pterygomaxillary fossa, a lateral rhinotomy combined with a Cadwell-Luc incision and transpalatine approach provides excellent exposure to all of the anatomic areas involved. Preoperative arterial embolization of the tumor through the external carotid artery has been a useful approach in some instances from the standpoint of reducing intraoperative hemorrhage (18). Freezing the lesion prior to resection has been used with a similar purpose.

The value of radiation therapy in the control of these tumors is still undetermined. It has been used as an adjuvant to the surgical approach, either as a preoperative measure to induce regression of large tumors, or postoperatively when operative removal has been incomplete. The usual dose is 3000–4000 rads in three weeks (8). Symptomatic relief is seen almost immediately, but the bulk of the tumor will take several months to reduce. The use of radiation therapy in children is not favored because of the potential of additional neoplastic change (5).

Summary

There are some unique soft-tissue tumors in the head and neck region, but generally this is an uncommon site for soft-tissue sarcomas in the adult population. Most of the surgical principles involved in the management of these lesions in the head and neck are quite similar to those described for other anatomic sites, but both the proximity of vital structures and the cosmetic deformities associated with operation produce special problems for the head and neck surgeon.

References

 1. Ariyan S: Further experiences with the pectoralis major myocutaneous flap for the immediate repair of defects from excisions of head and neck cancers. Plast Reconstr Surg 64:604–612, 1979.
 2. Bailey BJ, Barton S: Olfactory neuroblastoma: management and prognosis. Arch Otolaryngol 101:1–5, 1975.
 3. Biller HF III, Sessions DG, Ogura JH: Angiofibroma: a treatment approach. Laryngoscope 84:695–706, 1974.
 4. Boles R, Dedo H: Nasopharyngeal angiofibroma. Laryngoscope 5:364–372, 1976.
 5. Chen KT, Bauer FW: Sarcomatous transformation of nasopharyngeal angiofibroma. Cancer 49:369–371, 1982.
 6. Dial P, Marks C, Bolton J: Current management of paragangliomas. Surg Gynecol Obstet 155:187–192, 1982.
 7. Farr HW: Soft part sarcomas of the head and neck. Semin Oncol 8:185–189, 1981.
 8. Fitzpatrick PJ, Rider WD: The radiotherapy of nasopharyngeal angiofibroma. Radiology 109:171–178, 1973.
 9. Fu YS, Perzin KH: Non-epithelial tumors of the nasal cavity, paranasal sinuses and nasopharynx: a clinicopathologic study. I. General features and vascular tumors. Cancer 33:1275–1288, 1974.
10. Guillamondegui OM, Larson DL: The lateral trapezius musculocutaneous flap: its use in head and neck reconstruction. Plast Reconstr Surg 67:143–150, 1981.
11. Hatfield FP, James AE, Schulz MD: Chemodectomas of the glomus jugulare. Cancer 30:1164–1168, 1972.
12. Hutter RVP, Lewis JS, Foote FW: Esthesioneuroblastoma: a clinical and pathological study. Am J Surg 106:748–753, 1963.
13. Krupski WC, Effeney DJ, Ehrenfield WK, Stoney RJ: Cervical chemodectoma (technical considerations and management options). Am J Surg 144:215–220, 1982.

14. Lee DA, Rao BR, Meyer JS, et al: Hormonal receptor determination in juvenile nasopharyngeal angiofibromas. Cancer 46:547–551, 1980.
15. Mathes SJ, Nahai F: Clinical Applications for Muscle and Musculocutaneous Flaps. St Louis, CV Mosby, 1982.
16. Murphy TE, Huvos AF, Frazell EL: Chemodectomas of the glomus intravagale: vagal body tumors, nonchromaffin paragangliomas of the nodose ganglion of the vagus nerve. Ann Surg 172:246–255, 1970.
17. Neel HB III, Whicker JH, Devine KD, et al: Juvenile angiofibroma: review of 120 cases. Am J Surg 126:547–556, 1973.
18. Pletcher JD, Newton JH, Dedo HH, et al: Preoperative embolization of juvenile angiofibromas of nasopharynx. Ann Otol 84:740–746, 1975.
19. Shamblin WR, ReMine WH, Sheps GS, Harrison EG Jr: Carotid body tumor (chemodectoma): clinicopathological analysis of 90 cases. Am J Surg 124:510–514, 1971.
20. Shmookler BM, Enzinger FM, Brannon RB: Orofacial synovial sarcoma. Cancer 50:269–276, 1982.
21. Spector GJ, Maisel RH, Ogura JH: Glomus tumors in the middle ear: I. An analysis of 46 patients. Laryngoscope 83:1652–1672, 1973.

9 Musculocutaneous Flaps in Reconstruction

A well-planned repair of anatomic defects following appropriate surgical procedures for soft-tissue sarcoma facilitates prompt functional and physical rehabilitation of the patient, minimizes the morbidity associated with the loss of tissue, and effectively decreases the duration of hospitalization. Most surgical defects can be successfully repaired by the mobilization of local flaps or the judicious use of skin grafts. However, the removal of large tumors of the trunk, abdominal wall, and extremities may result in full-thickness defects in the chest, abdomen, perineum, or expose bones or neurovascular structures in the extremities. The lack of familiarity with modern reconstructive procedures has led inexperienced surgeons to resort to alternative, less than optimal forms of therapy of the primary sarcoma (chemotherapy, radiotherapy, or amputation) with resultant inadequate tumor control in many instances or significant functional and physical disability. The extensive experience accumulated in the past decade with the transposition and free grafting of musculocutaneous flaps has led to primary and effective reconstruction of many of these surgical defects. It has also allowed new techniques for limb preservation by providing viable and functional coverage for vital limb structures (neurovascular supply, bone, joints) following the adequate resection of soft-tissue sarcomas.

General Principles

The musculocutaneous flap is a unit of muscle with overlying skin which derives its blood supply from a well-identified vascular pedicle to the muscle; the muscle acts as a carrier of the cutaneous segment, which is vascularized by perforant vessels from the underlying muscle. This island of skin can be designed to fit the shape and size of the surgical defect. Additional skin surface can be obtained by extending the skin flap (up to one-third of the total area) beyond the muscle; however, this portion of skin beyond the underlying muscle base has a random blood supply, which is derived from subfascial or dermal vessels, and its viability is not as certain.

The musculocutaneous flap, once detached from its muscular insertion, has a wide arc of rotation, with its vascular pedicle determining the mobility or the axis of rotation. Furthermore, the entire flap may be transferred as a free flap by means of microvascular anastomoses, but this depends on the

150

number, location, and variations in the vessels in the vascular pedicle to the muscle (4,6–8).

Most of the major muscles have a vascular communication with periosteum at the site of bone insertion. This segment of bone, when located distal to the point of rotation, can be incorporated with the musculocutaneous unit when bone replacement is indicated (e.g., rib or sternum with pectoralis major muscle for mandibular reconstruction). The viability, versatility of design of the musculocutaneous flap, and final physical and functional results are mostly dependent on the surgeon's knowledge of the anatomic location and distribution of the blood supply to the selected muscle. Division of the nerve supply to the muscle will result in its progressive atrophy, reducing significantly its original size if the bulk of the muscle tissue is not required as part of the reconstruction. The flap donor site usually can be closed primarily, leaving a minimal defect. Once the musculocutaneous unit has been raised, it can be tunneled without difficulty under the bridge of skin that may separate the donor from the recipient site.

Surgical Anatomy

The most common defects in the head and neck, trunk, perineum, and proximal extremities can be successfully repaired with the transposition of regional muscle flaps. However, certain defects in the skull or distal extremities may require the use of microvascular techniques for optimal functional and cosmetic results.

We will briefly outline the most pertinent features of the commonly used musculocutaneous flaps (Table 9-1 and Fig. 9-1). For more detailed descriptions, the reader should consult articles in the bibliography (3,6,7).

Latissimus Dorsi
Transposition of the latissimus dorsi flap will cover anterior and lateral chest wall, axilla, interscapular area, and shoulder defects, major defects of the arm, head, and neck, and is especially useful for reconstruction in the breast and pectoral region.

This muscle derives its blood supply from the thoracodorsal artery (branch of the subscapular artery), which arises from the lateral third of the axillary artery and enters the deep surface of the muscle high in the axilla. Perforant vessels from dorsal branches of the last seven intercostal spaces and four lumbar arteries will allow the transposition of the latissimus

Table 9-1. Flap Selection for Different Anatomic Areas

Head and neck	Muscles
Oral cavity	
Pharynx	Pectoralis major
Face, temporal region	Upper trapezius
Posterior neck	
Occipital region	Upper and lower trapezius
Chest and shoulder	Pectoralis major
	Latissimus dorsi
	Rectus abdominis
Abdomen, groin, and perineum	Rectus abdominis
	Tensor fascia lata
	Gracilis
	Sartorius

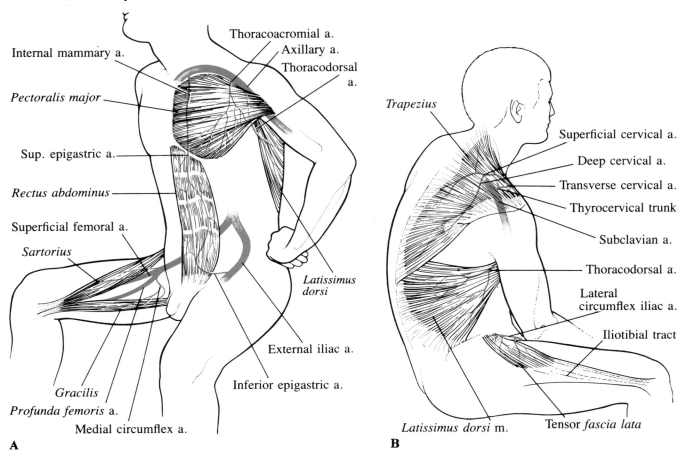

FIG. 9-1. A and **B.** Location of the most commonly utilized musculocutaneous flaps. The arterial blood supply to these muscles is illustrated; their arc of rotation can be inferred from the vascular origin and is described in the text.

dorsi flap in reverse fashion when this is indicated. An example of this flap for reconstruction of a chest wall defect is shown in Figure 9-2.

Pectoralis Major

The pectoralis major has played a major role in reconstruction of most areas in the head and neck (1) (external covering for neck, face, temporal area, floor of the mouth, tongue, partial and total pharyngectomy, and for primary reconstruction of the cervical esophagus). In addition, it can be used for coverage of the shoulder (Fig. 9-3) and for contralateral chest wall defects. Vascular communication with the underlying periosteum allows this muscle to carry a segment of rib or sternum for mandibular reconstruction (2,7).

The predominant blood supply for this flap is the pectoral branch of the thoracoacromial artery, a branch of the axillary artery, which runs along the deep surface of the pectoralis major muscle in association with the lateral thoracic nerve. The secondary vessels are those from the first to sixth intercostal spaces. The pectoral branch of the thoracoacromial artery constitutes the axis of transposition of the muscle pedicle. The remaining vessels can be divided without interfering with the viability of the flap. The island of skin can be outlined medial or inferior to the nipple and extended over the rectus fascia (random portion) if needed.

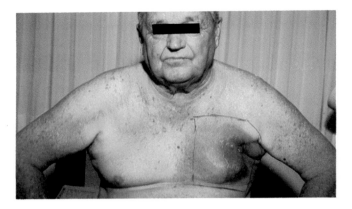

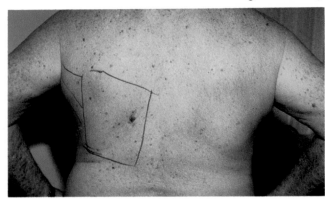

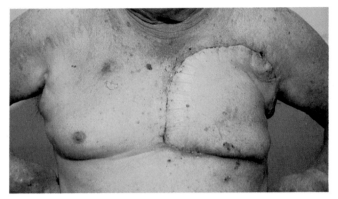

A

B

FIG. 9-2. **A.** Recurrent liposarcoma of the anterior chest wall following radiotherapy. The proposed resection is outlined. **B.** Outline of the latissimus dorsi flap. In this case the flap is based anteriorly on the thoracodorsal vessels. **C.** Postoperative view.

C

Trapezius

The predominant blood supply of the trapezius flap is the transverse cervical artery, a branch of the thyrocervical trunk. This artery runs parallel to the clavicle between the brachial plexus and anterior scalene muscle and the omohyoid muscle. After reaching the trapezius, the transverse cervical artery divides into a superficial branch, which supplies the upper trapezius, and a deep branch, which runs posteriorly along the deep surface of the lower two-thirds of the trapezius. The spine of the scapula separates the upper from the lower trapezius (5).

The upper trapezius flap can carry an island of skin from the anterior border of the trapezius to the spine of the scapula. Laterally, the skin flap can be extended beyond the acromioclavicular joint over the deltoid muscle (random portion). After the island of skin is delineated, the transverse cervical artery is identified in the supraclavicular region and traced along the undersurface of the upper trapezius. The upper trapezius flap is separated from the lower trapezius along the superior border of the spine of the scapula and from its clavicular and acromial insertions. The myocutaneous unit is then elevated, preserving its vascular supply and the spinal accessory nerve; the proximal segment of the muscle is divided from its occipital insertion. This flap can cover most defects of the neck, temporal-occipital, maxillofacial, and oropharyngeal areas.

The lower part of the trapezius can carry the skin along the scapulospinal region. After the skin island is outlined, the myocutaneous unit is raised from the sacrospinalis muscle and detached from the thoracic spinal processes and spine of the scapula. The trapezius is then divided from its upper segment

153

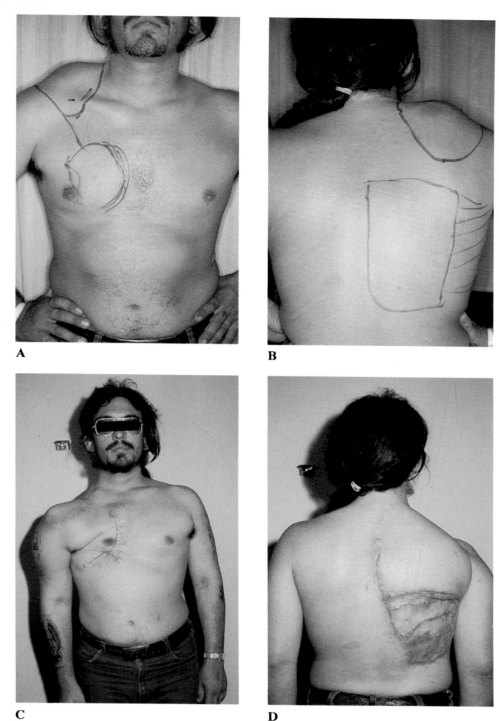

A

B

C

D

FIG. 9-3. **A,B.** Malignant schwannoma involving the scapula. Anterior and posterior views demonstrating the area of proposed resection (*above*), including total scapulectomy, and proposed reconstruction using pectoralis major musculocutaneous (**A**) and latissimus dorsi musculocutaneous (**B**) flaps. **C,D.** Postoperative views.

above the spine of the scapula and is rotated to the designated area. Lower trapezius myocutaneous flaps will cover defects in the posterior neck, occipital-temporal, and zygomatic areas.

Rectus Abdominis

The rectus abdominis obtains its blood supply from the superior epigastric artery (an extension of the internal mammary), which emerges from under the costal margin and runs along the posterior surface of the muscle to join the inferior epigastric artery (which arises from the external iliac artery).

154

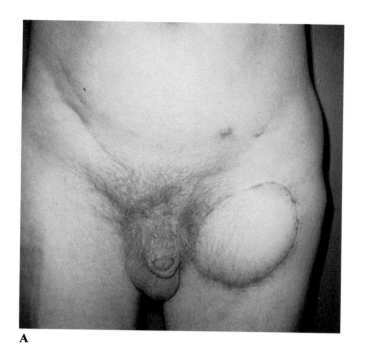
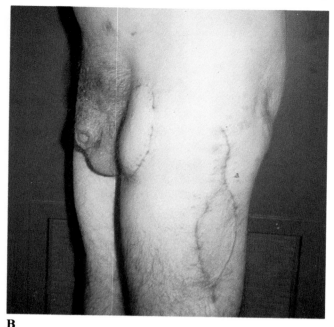

A

B

FIG. 9-4. **A.** Postoperative view of tensor fascia lata musculocutaneous flap utilized to cover a groin defect following resection of a synovial sarcoma. **B.** Donor site of same patient.

This double pedicle allows the use of the flap in two different axes. The superior axis facilitates coverage of anterior and lateral chest wall defects and the inferior axis of rotation will cover defects in the groin, pubis, perineum, lateral flank, and pelvis (3).

Tensor Fascia Lata

The tensor fascia lata arises from the anterior third of the anterior iliac spine, overlies the gluteus medius and proximal sartorius, and blends with the iliotibial tract. The predominant vascular supply is the lateral circumflex iliac artery, a branch of the profunda femoris, which emerges from behind the rectus femoris and enters the tensor fascia lata muscle in its upper third, about 6 cm below the anterior iliac spine. This vessel then runs parallel to the fascia lata and sends perforators to the skin. These perforators supply the skin in the anterolateral mid and lower thigh beyond the muscle itself. After the island of skin is outlined, the fascia lata is divided inferiorly at the level of the lateral condyle. The flap is raised anteriorly and posteriorly from the vastus lateralis and will cover defects in the perineum, sacral area, groin (Fig. 9-4), pubic area, and lower abdominal wall. A skin graft will usually be necessary to cover the donor site. Vascular communication with the periosteum of the anterior iliac spine allows the inclusion of bone in free transplants (3).

Sartorius

The sartorius arises from the anterior iliac spine, extends medially across the thigh, and inserts near the knee on the medial surface of the upper tibia with the gracilis and semitendinosus muscles. The blood supply derives from multiple segmental muscular branches of the common femoral artery. The flap will cover the perineum (Fig. 9-5), pubic area, and defects in the medial aspect of the thigh and groin (3–6).

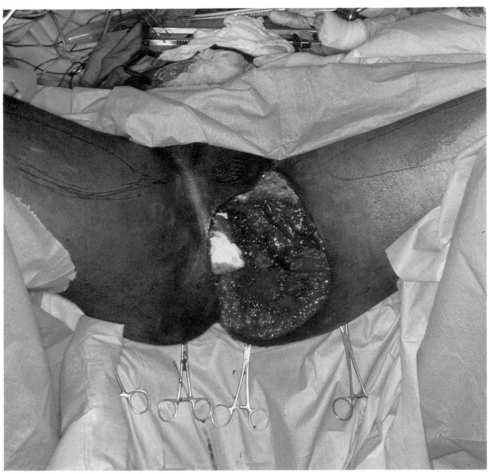

FIG. 9-5. **A.** Postoperative view following total pelvic exenteration with resection of perineum and left ischiopubic ramus for rhabdomyosarcoma. **B,C.** Sartorius (*left*) and gracilis (*right*) musculocutaneous flaps were transposed for perineal repair.

A

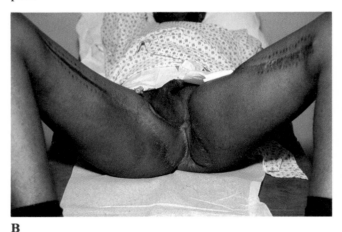

B

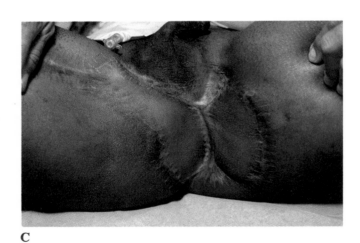

C

Gracilis

The gracilis arises from the ischiopubic bone and inserts distally in the proximal tibia with the sartorius and semitendinosus. Its blood supply arises from medial circumflex branches of the profunda femoris artery and reaches the muscle 8 to 10 cm below the proximal insertion between the adductor longus and brevis. This flap has gained significant popularity in gynecologic oncology for vaginal and perineal reconstruction (Fig. 9-5) following total pelvic exenteration with wide resection of the perineum.

Complications

The viability of musculocutaneous flaps depends primarily on preservation of arterial flow to and venous flow from the muscle tissue that is utilized as a carrier for the overlying skin. Injury to these vessels, or interference with flow produced by acute angulation of the vascular pedicle, may lead to necrosis of all or part of the muscle and the overlying skin. Thus, great care must be taken to preserve the key vessels nourishing the musculocutaneous flap. Also, the vascularity of the skin should be carefully observed after the rotation of the muscle and its pedicle have been accomplished. It may be necessary to return the flap to its original bed, or more often the flap rotation may be modified so as to maintain adequate circulation.

Another cause of total or partial skin loss with a musculocutaneous flap is the failure to preserve the vessels feeding the flap from the underlying muscle. A modification of this mechanism of skin loss may result from too great an extension of the skin flap past the limits of the underlying muscle, the so-called random portion of the flap. Necrosis of this portion of the skin flap, the part nourished from the adjacent skin, is not rare. This complication may seriously jeopardize the reconstruction, prolong the hospital stay, increase the long-term morbidity, and adversely affect the ultimate cosmetic result.

Fluid collections, particularly blood and serum, often occur in the wound of the donor site of a musculocutaneous flap. This is adequate justification for closed suction tube drainage of these wounds, which is usually required for several days. Some of these same sites, closed under tension, may break down or demonstrate wound separation. All of these potential complications are relatively uncommon and can be minimized by attention to details throughout the reconstruction.

References

1. Ariyan S: Further experiences with the *pectoralis major* myocutaneous flap for the immediate repair of defects from excisions of head and neck cancers. Plast Reconstr Surg 64:605–612, 1979.
2. Arnold PG, Pairolero PC: Use of *pectoralis major* muscle flaps to repair defects of anterior chest wall. Plast Reconstr Surg 63:205–213, 1979.
3. Bostwick J III, Hill HL, Nahai F: Repairs in the lower abdomen, groin, or perineum with myocutaneous or omental flaps. Plast Reconstr Surg 63:186–194, 1979.
4. Daniel RK, Taylor GI: Distant transfer of an island flap by microvascular anastomoses. Plast Reconstr Surg 52:111–117, 1973.
5. Guillamondegui OM, Larson DL: The lateral trapezius musculocutaneous flap: Its use in head and neck reconstruction. Plast Reconstr Surg 67:143–150, 1981.
6. McCraw JB, Dibbel DG, Carraway JH: Clinical definition of independent myocutaneous vascular territories. Plast Reconstr Surg 60:341–352, 1977.
7. Mathes SJ, Nahai F: Clinical Applications for Muscle and Musculocutaneous Flaps. St. Louis, Missouri, CV Mosby Company, 1982.
8. Taylor GI, Daniel RK: The anatomy of several free flap donor sites. Plast Reconstr Surg 56:243–253, 1975.

10 Rehabilitation of the Sarcoma Patient

The surgical management of soft-tissue sarcoma is not infrequently associated with various degrees of physical disability, which may range from limitation in range of motion to loss of an extremity. The loss of function may result in discomfort from prolonged sitting, standing, and walking, difficulty in running or kneeling, precarious balance, restrictions in lifting, and inability to hold or grasp objects. The fear of the anticipated disability from treatment produces significant anxiety in the patient and his family, with major concerns of dependence, pain, alteration of self-image, loss of self-esteem, and psychosexual adjustment problems. A well-planned program for rehabilitation will minimize the psychosocial and functional impact of any loss of function from treatment by restoring the patient to self-sufficiency at his highest attainable skill in the shortest period of time. These goals are attained optimally through early intervention of a multidisciplinary team integrated by the surgeon which should include a physical medicine specialist (physiatrist), social worker, nurse, psychologist, occupational and physical therapists, and a vocational rehabilitation counselor.

The process of rehabilitation starts with the initial assessment of the extent of surgery and a psychosocial profile of the patient and the immediate family. The surgeon will discuss the importance of the planned procedure to assure control of the sarcoma, and must convey a true picture of the physical and functional disability that may result from the proposed treatment. At this time the rehabilitation program is also discussed, pointing out the positive aspects of the recovery period, outlining the expected recovery from initial loss of function and compensatory means for dealing with the permanent disability (brace, prosthesis, etc.), the probability of continuing with preillness performance, and available alternatives. Subsequent meetings between the patient and different members of the rehabilitation team will facilitate understanding of the treatment plan and the outlook for recovery as well as making the patient and his family full participants in the recovery process. With the current emphasis on adjuvant therapy programs and limb-saving procedures, a significant number of patients with soft-tissue sarcomas will receive radiotherapy and/or chemotherapy as part of their initial therapy. Both the importance and possible side effects of these therapeutic modalities should be explained to the patient, but other therapy should not be allowed to delay the implementation of the rehabilitation program.

Principles of Physical Rehabilitation

Soft-Part Resection

The rehabilitation of the functional deficit resulting from resection of the muscle surrounding a sarcoma is based on the development of appropriate compensatory function from adjacent muscle groups and the use of selected external devices (braces) to obtain maximal performance by the affected limb. All soft-part resections on the extremities are procedures that are being employed in lieu of amputation. The patient usually has a very positive attitude toward physical rehabilitation after operation, since he (or she) knows that "limb salvage" has been achieved. Some degree of persisting disability is well accepted, since amputation was the alternative.

Lower Extremity: Resection of the buttock muscles weakens extension of the hip and external rotation of the thigh. The act of stair climbing or rising from a sitting position is also impaired by this procedure. Training is directed toward dependence upon the uninvolved lower extremity for provision of compensatory function. The resection of the hamstring or quadriceps muscle group interferes with flexion or extension, respectively, of the leg. Climbing, rising, and running are hampered by these operations. The use of a knee brace, active physical therapy of the residual muscle groups, and gait training will correct most of the early motor disabilities, leaving running as the major residual handicap. Deficits from resection of the gastrocnemius and soleus or anterior tibial compartment muscles (toe stubbing, tripping) are corrected with the use of an ankle brace and gait training. In all of these situations the patient usually develops enough strength in residual musculature over time to discontinue the use of the brace (Fig. 10-1).

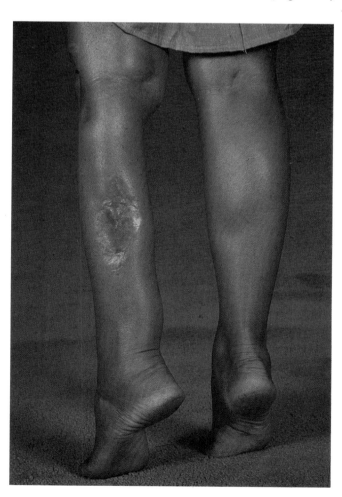

FIG. 10-1. Patient who is one year postoperative after soft-tissue resection of a sarcoma arising in the calf musculature. The entire gastrocnemius and soleus were resected (see Fig. 5-31). The efficiency of plantar flexion by means of the posterior tibialis muscle is well demonstrated in this patient, who is able to walk normally as well as being able to stand on her toes, as shown.

159

Upper Extremity: Resection of the shoulder girdle (scapulectomy, Tikhoff-Linberg procedure) preserves the physical integrity of the upper extremity and the function of the forearm and hand. However, the patient loses the normal functions of the shoulder and elbow. With the Tikhoff-Linberg procedure the arm is attached to the trunk only by skin and the neurovascular bundle, and this places significant strain on the brachial plexus. A properly constructed brace placed around the waist before this operation will support the elbow at a functional level, thereby allowing the full use of the forearm and hand. Alternatively, a metallic interpositional device inserted operatively can be used to fix the humerus to the second rib, thus increasing stability and function (5).

When an anterior or posterior compartmental resection is performed for a sarcoma arising on the upper arm, the major functional disability is that of defective elbow function. Compensation depends on effective use of the force of gravity. For those lesions requiring radial nerve resection, the resulting wristdrop can be managed by a brace or splint, but subsequent tendon transfers should provide excellent function and maintain the wrist in a position of function. The resection of volar or extensor muscle groups in the forearm produces a deficit in wrist and hand function. The use of dynamic or active splinting for the distal hand and wrist gives the patient's joints mobility and directional control, and this substitutes for the absence of muscle power. The proper use of these splints helps maintain normal joint function in one hand.

Amputations

The prospect of amputation uniformly provokes significant anxiety in the patient, as there is fear of the crippling effects as well as the loss of self-esteem and independence. Careful explanation of the actual degree of disability, an outline of the rehabilitation program designed to compensate for the lost limb, and a social visit from a cancer amputee are extremely useful in dispelling these apprehensions. As part of the preoperative discussion, the patient also should be made aware of postoperative "phantom" sensations and reassured regarding their eventual adjustments.

Lower Extremity: Prosthetic rehabilitation of the lower limb amputee starts with the construction of the stump. A proper myoplasty, securing the muscles over the bone, ensures a well-protected stump, allows control of movement by the attached muscles, and results in a well-functioning prosthesis. A plaster of paris dressing wrapped around the stump will prevent edema and also allows the application of an immediate temporary prosthesis for early ambulation. At 14 days the plaster can be removed for stump inspection, the removal of sutures, and patient instruction in care of the stump. After 4 to 6 weeks arrangements for a permanent prosthesis can be made.

The level of amputation determines the degree of functional recovery that may be expected. Patients undergoing hemipelvectomy or hip joint disarticulation will never have as satisfactory a functional and cosmetic result as those having amputations at a more distal level. The higher the level of amputation, the more cumbersome the prosthesis, the longer the training period, and the greater the energy expended on its use. Well-trained amputees with hemipelvectomy or hip joint disarticulation usually ambulate more efficiently with crutches than with their prosthesis (Fig. 10-2).

The Hand: The length of fingers and hand should be preserved with some exceptions. In amputation of phalanges, it is better to shorten the finger slightly than to leave the bulbous and distal expansion of these bones. The distal two-thirds of the second, third, fourth, and fifth metacarpals should be excised when the corresponding fingers are sacrificed; these knuckles, in

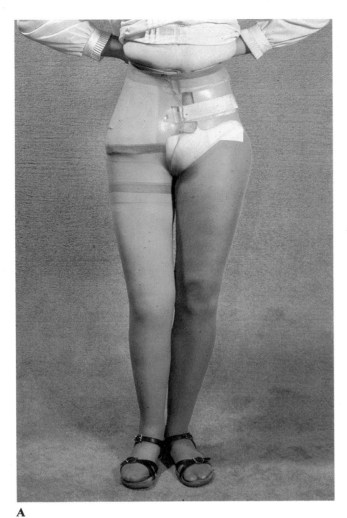 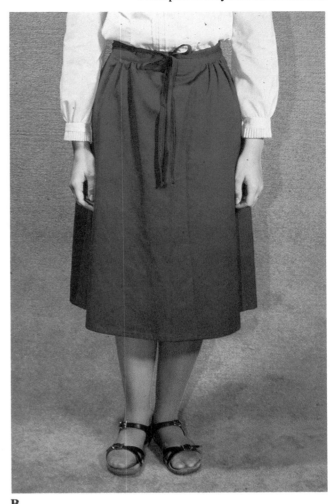

A   B

FIG. 10-2. **A** and **B.** The prosthesis utilized by a patient following hemipelvectomy allows her to walk without a cane. Considerable rehabilitative effort is required to achieve reasonable function with this prosthesis.

the absence of fingers, are unsightly and the skin is sensitive and traumatized frequently. This also allows the fingers to be closer together and, therefore, in a better position for function.

Wrist and Forearm: Amputation through the wrist can be well fitted with a wrist disarticulation prosthesis which allows dorsal and volar flexion and full rotation while providing a functional prehensive device. For these amputations, the radial and ulnar styloid should be removed for better tolerance and function of the prosthesis.

Amputation at and Above the Elbow: Newer devices, such as step-up elbow hinges and outside-locking elbow joints, have overcome technical difficulties associated with construction of a prosthesis to be applied around an amputation close to the elbow. With amputations above the elbow, all possible bone length should be preserved. Although the humeral stump above the deltoid and pectoral insertions lacks motion, every inch distal is functional and increases the stability and function of an arm prosthesis.

Patients undergoing shoulder disarticulation or interscapulothoracic amputation are not generally candidates for prostheses for technical reasons. A

161

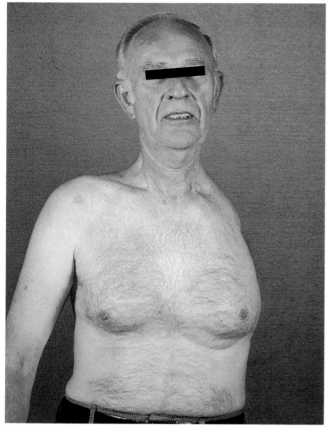

A

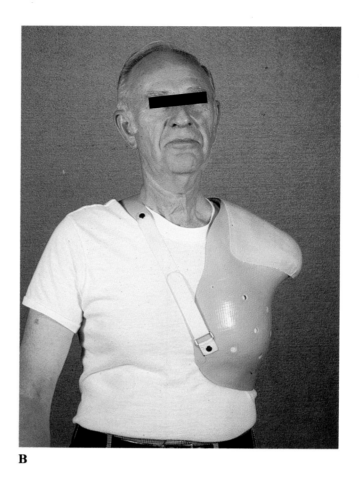

B

FIG. 10-3. This patient who has been treated by inter-scapulothoracic amputation has a major deformity that is demonstrated in **A.** The prosthetic shoulder cap prosthesis **(B)** allows proper fit for his clothing **(C).**

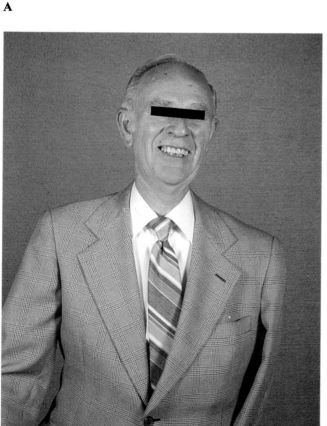

C

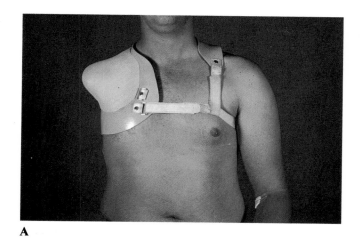
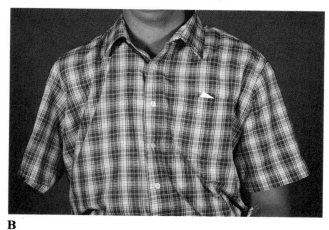

A   B

FIG. 10-4. **A** and **B.** A variation in shoulder cap prosthesis for the purpose of a natural appearance when dressed despite the absent upper extremity.

well-built shoulder cap supports clothing and enhances cosmetic appearance (Figs. 10-3 and 10-4). Those patients utilizing a substitute-arm prosthesis after interscapulothoracic amputation wear this more for appearance than function.

References

1. Dietz JH Jr: Rehabilitation Oncology. New York, John Wiley & Sons, 1981.
2. Malick MH: Manual on Dynamic Hand Splinting with Thermoplastic Materials. Hamarville Rehabilitation Center, 1974.
3. National Cancer Institute Monograph 56: Sarcomas of Soft Tissue and Bone in Childhood, April 1981.
4. Santschi WR: Manual of Upper Extremity Prosthetics. University of California at Los Angeles, 1958.
5. Whitehill R, Wanebo HJ, Mabie KN, Schildwachter T, Rosenberger R: Reconstruction after the Tikhoff-Linberg procedure. Arch Surg 117:1248–1249, 1982.

Additional Considerations in Sarcoma Management

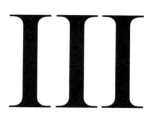

Adjuvant Therapy for Sarcomas in Adults

11

The treatment considered optimal for primary soft-tissue sarcomas is operative resection with adequate margins of normal tissue around the neoplasm. This approach has been fully illustrated earlier in this volume for a variety of primary sites and clinical presentations. With this approach, the overall "cure rate" for localized soft-tissue sarcomas in adults has been in the range of 40%. More recent reports do suggest a somewhat higher figure, but this may be due to better initial staging methods and the resulting separation of patients with clinically unsuspected metastatic disease. Unfortunately, local control of the sarcoma is not always achieved by operative resection, despite an attempt to follow the surgical principles that have been outlined. In some instances, local failure may occur due to employment of a less than radical approach in order to maintain a viable extremity or because of other anatomic limitations associated with sarcomas arising from the trunk, retroperitoneum, or the head and neck. Nonoperative adjuvant therapies have been employed to deal with both problems associated with treatment failure—local recurrence and hematogenous metastases. An attempt will be made to assess the value of these additional approaches to clinical management.

Radiation as Potential Adjuvant Therapy

In a 25-year retrospective evaluation, McNeer and coauthors (13) in 1968 reported that soft-tissue sarcomas could occasionally be cured by radiation therapy alone and that radiation therapy administered as an adjuvant to surgery could improve "cure rates" for some sarcomas when compared with results from surgery alone. The patients reported in this series were not randomized, the doses of radiation employed were quite variable, and prognostic variables such as size, primary site, or degree of differentiation were not considered in the assessment. An important finding, however, was that 42 of 58 patients (72%) suitable for complete clinical evaluation after preoperative radiation or radiation as the only treatment had objective regression in tumor size, and 24 of the total 72 patients (33%) treated had a complete local response to radiation treatment alone. Thus, this report provided the background for later, more intensive preoperative or postoperative radiation therapy regimes utilized in an attempt to improve local control rates. The authors expressed the need for a prospective trial of combined radiation and adequate operative treatment, but a controlled trial specifically designed to assess the role of radiation after "radical" surgery for adult sarcomas has not yet been performed.

Reports by Lindberg and others from the M. D. Anderson Hospital and Tumor Institute (7,8,21–23) have described the use of high-dose radiation therapy following conservative surgical excision of soft-tissue sarcomas. All patients in this series were 16 years of age or older, had no evidence of metastatic sarcoma on admission, underwent total excision of the tumor mass (with or without "negative" margins), and received at least 5000 rads in 5 weeks following surgery; patients receiving less than 5000 rads in 5 weeks were not included. An unknown number of patients were thereby excluded; reported results were based on 300 patients with at least a 2-year follow-up, 168 of whom were available for at least a 5-year follow-up.

Radiation therapy was begun within 3–4 weeks of the surgical resection and, for extremity tumors, included the entire surgical field with a 5–7 cm margin. Initially, patients received 7000–7500 rads with a shrinking field technique after 5000 rads; later a total dose of 6000–6500 rads was administered and, whenever possible, less than one-half the cross section of the extremity was irradiated to reduce the possibility of subsequent edema.

The 2-year disease-free survival in this series was 74% (222 of 300). Eighteen of the 222 patients who were disease-free 2 years later had local recurrence but were tumor-free following subsequent surgery; 21 (7%) subsequently died with local recurrence at the primary site and 55 (18.3%) died with distant metastases but maintained local control at the primary site. Of the 67 patients with local recurrence following combined treatment, 32 of 40 were controlled by a subsequent surgical effort (11 wide excisions, 21 amputations). The 5-year disease-free survival for the entire series was 61.3% (103 of 168). Overall, 67% of local recurrences became apparent within 2 years of treatment and 92.5% within 5 years. Five additional patients developed local recurrence after the 5-year interval. Thus, the overall incidence of local recurrences of 22.5% is likely to increase when all treated patients have been followed for the full 5 years.

When local recurrence rates were correlated with primary tumor site, several points became evident. Upper extremity tumors had fewer local recurrences (10 of 63, or 15.9%) than intraabdominal tumors (8 of 21, or 38.1%), and the rate of distant metastases correlated with rates of local recurrence. Although an earlier report (7) had suggested local recurrences were more common in proximal extremity tumors, this did not remain true with a larger series of patients (8). When histologic diagnosis was correlated with local recurrence rate, liposarcomas (5 of 41) and fibrosarcomas (5 of 41) had the best local control rates, but neurofibrosarcomas (20 of 60) had the worst. Although one would expect size to be an important prognostic variable in determining local recurrence, this appeared to be true only for grade II tumors; patients with grade I tumors did uniformly well despite the size of the primary tumor, and patients with grade III tumors had high local recurrence rates even with primary tumors less than 5 cm in size.

Significant complications occurred in 13 of 200 patients (6.5%) with extremity tumors: these included soft-tissue necrosis, fracture, impaired motion, neurovascular damage, and edema. One patient required amputation for extensive soft-tissue damage. The great majority of extremity sarcoma patients, therefore, had a functional limb preserved, and disease-free survival rates were quite similar to those obtained in most purely surgical series.

These retrospective data from the M. D. Anderson Hospital suggest that conservative surgery combined with postoperative radiation therapy is as efficacious in controlling the local disease as is radical surgery without radiation. However, several problems remain unresolved. First, the reported patients were treated over a long period of time, yet 43% were available for only 2-year follow-up; further follow-up information may show increasing local recurrence rates. Second, an unknown number of patients were excluded from analysis because they did not (could not?) receive 5000 rads in 5 weeks. Third, the authors did not describe in detail the operations performed; they state a "limited amount of normal tissue" was resected with the tumor (8), but this was not defined. It would be important to know if patients with histologically involved margins had a higher local recurrence rate than patients with histologically negative margins, as suggested by Rosenberg (15). Patients with inadequate margins might benefit from amputation rather than conservative efforts to attempt limb preservation. Last, but not least, the retrospective nonrandomized nature of the observations makes accurate comparison impossible between the results obtained with conservative surgery and postoperative irradiation and those obtained with adequate surgery alone.

A randomized, prospective trial comparing conservative surgery followed by radiation (4500–5000 rads followed by a shrinking field technique to boost the tumor bed dose to 6000–7000 rads) with amputation has been performed by the Surgery and Radiation Oncology Branches of the National Cancer Institute (15–18). All patients also received adjuvant chemotherapy (adriamycin and cyclophosphamide). In patients undergoing conservative resection followed by radiation therapy, there were 3 local recurrences among 8 patients with positive margins, but no local recurrences among 44 patients with negative surgical margins ($p < 0.0001$); none of the patients with amputations developed local recurrence. The role of adjuvant chemotherapy was assessed in a later trial, but the authors suggested that a microscopically positive margin might be an indication for secondary amputation.

Suit and his co-workers from the Massachusetts General Hospital (20) have reported a series of 36 patients treated preoperatively by radiation therapy (generally 5000–6000 rads) followed two weeks later by attempted conservative resection with either an intraoperative boost to the tumor bed or additional radiation therapy given postoperatively. Seven of these patients could not have a conservative resection performed: 4 required amputation, and 3 had major involvement of neurovascular structures and had their primary treatment completed by radiation therapy. Findings from this study included a greater effect on the histology of the sarcoma with increasing dosage of radiation, especially when this was above 4000 rads. Among 28 patients followed for over one year, 24 of 25 patients undergoing subsequent resection maintained local control of their tumor, but 10 of these patients developed distant metastases; 1 of 3 patients, who was not resected and received additional radiotherapy, had local control, and the other 2 patients developed distant metastases. Delays in wound healing were found in 6 of 33 patients who underwent resection following radiation therapy. These data suggest that aggressive preoperative and perioperative radiation therapy, accompanied by conservative operations, is reasonably effective in obtaining local tumor control, but it was striking that many tumors in this study were relatively small (18 were stage I or II, and 15 were stage III). Conclusions regarding the benefits of preoperative radiation must be tempered by this fact.

These data from several sources all suggest that conservative surgery prior to or following radiation therapy may control local, resectable adult sarcomas as effectively as surgical resection alone. However, because these same sarcomas have low recurrence rates if truly adequate soft-part resections are performed (and, therefore, a functional limb preserved), the question still

169

remains as to whether radiation therapy actually improves local control over that obtained by adequate surgery alone. Neither the retrospective reviews nor the single randomized trial comparing a conservative approach with amputation have really settled the issue.

The only prospective randomized trial of adjuvant radiation when adequate margins were achieved for sarcomas is the Intergroup Rhabdomyosarcoma Study of postoperative radiation for childhood rhabdomyosarcoma. In this study postoperative radiation did not affect either local or distant recurrence rates (see Chapter 13). This same experiment must be performed in adult sarcoma patients to convincingly establish real benefit from adjuvant radiation in this clinical setting.

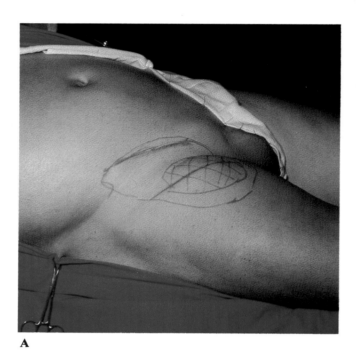

A

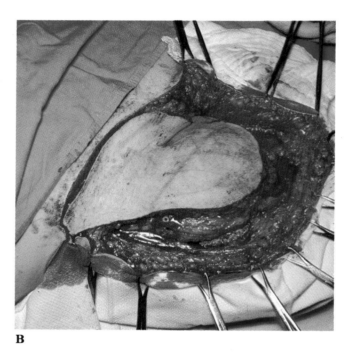

B

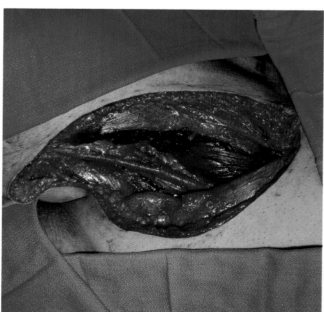

C

FIG. 11-1. Recurrent soft-tissue sarcoma in the groin area in a male patient who had previously been treated by "enucleation" **(A)**. Wide soft-tissue resection is planned, since hemipelvectomy is an unacceptable alternative to this patient. Wide resection of skin, subcutaneous tissue, and muscle over the region of the femoral triangle is demonstrated **(B)**. A narrow but clear soft-tissue margin was achieved with preservation of the femoral vessel as shown in this view of the completed dissection **(C)**. Closure was achieved by rotating an abdominal skin flap. Despite postoperative irradiation to the operative field, local recurrence became apparent five years later and necessitated hemipelvectomy at that time to achieve disease control.

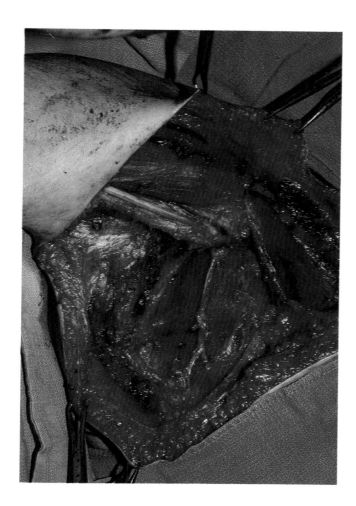

FIG. 11-2. Operative field after extensive soft-tissue resection for malignant fibrous histiocytoma of the axillary region arising from the teres major and latissimus dorsi muscles. The axillary neurovascular bundle seen in the operative wound had a clear but less than ideal margin of normal tissue, but limb preservation was achieved by the operation. This finding was considered an indication for postoperative irradiation as an adjuvant treatment.

It has been recommended that radiation be employed preoperatively or postoperatively for patients with microscopically high-grade sarcomas, particularly those treated by conservative procedures. The basis for this is the greater frequency of local recurrence after operative resection in this subpopulation of sarcoma patients. An advantage to the surgeon of postoperative radiation (over preoperative treatment) is the elimination of the problem of identifying the appropriate margin of resection at the time of operation. Preoperative therapy leading to gross reduction in the size of the sarcoma often makes determination of an appropriate surgical margin a difficult one. Although adding radiation to the treatment program in such selected patients (those with high-grade lesions) is a practical approach, particularly when a conservative excision is desired to avoid amputation (Fig. 11-1, 11-2), it does not seem wise to carry out operative procedures that do not achieve a clear margin. Radiation does not assure local control when the surgical margin is involved (15).

If adjuvant radiation therapy is eventually shown to improve the results obtained from truly adequate surgery, this would be important new information for future treatment planning. Hopefully, clinical trials will be completed in the future that clearly address this question. When the choice between amputation and more limited complete resection is presented, the proposal for adjuvant radiotherapy does seem reasonable on the basis of the data presented. In our practice adjuvant radiotherapy is employed for selected cases with high-grade lesions, while it is withheld from patients in whom truly adequate gross margins can be achieved by soft-part resection.

171

Adjuvant Chemotherapy

Since many patients with soft-tissue sarcomas succumb to metastatic disease despite local control, there have been some attempts to administer systemic therapy to try to prevent the subsequent appearance of metastases. The rationale for adjuvant chemotherapy has been recently reviewed by Martin (11). In brief, most cancer cells that are destroyed by chemotherapeutic drugs are killed via first-order kinetics; thus, no matter how many cancer cells are present, the same proportion is killed by each course of drugs. Accordingly, the optimal time to administer chemotherapy is when the total number of metastatic cancer cells is the smallest, i.e., soon after the operative resection of the primary lesion. Problems with such an approach include the possibility of drug resistance developing in the tumor cells that are not destroyed.

There are additional principles that are important in administering combination chemotherapy in the adjuvant setting. First, each drug used should have demonstrated activity against gross disease. Second, drugs utilized in combination regimens should have different mechanisms of action, and their individual toxicities should overlap as little as possible. Third, the chemotherapy should be administered at maximum tolerated dosages in intermittent courses, with the intervals between courses as short as possible. Fourth, the adjuvant chemotherapy program must be long enough to virtually eradicate the residual cancer cells.

Few studies have investigated the use of chemotherapy as an adjuvant to surgery (and/or radiation) for soft-tissue sarcomas, and fewer yet have done this in a prospective manner with a concomitant control group. Antman et al. (1) treated 19 patients with surgery, radiation, and chemotherapy (cyclophosphamide, adriamycin, and DTIC). The results were compared with those obtained in a group of sarcoma patients matched for stage and histology but treated without chemotherapy between 1954 and 1968. Patients receiving the combined-modality therapy had a significantly improved survival when compared with historical controls, but the treatment administered to the control patients was not reported. The authors used these pilot data as a basis for beginning a randomized, controlled trial, comparing a group of patients receiving chemotherapy to a group receiving no chemotherapy.

Das Gupta et al. compared a group of 113 patients receiving adriamycin and DTIC following surgical resection with 144 concurrently treated patients undergoing surgery alone (2). Staging, grading, anatomic location, and histologic types were similar in the two groups. Local recurrence rates were similar in both groups, but disease-free survival was higher in the group of patients receiving chemotherapy (77% versus 59% at 2 years and 74% versus 50% at 5 years). Most of the survival benefit appeared to be in those patients with malignant fibrous histiocytomas, leiomyosarcomas, or rhabdomyosarcomas. The authors, however, do not state why patients were selected to receive chemotherapy; more patients in the surgery-only group underwent amputation, thereby suggesting this group may have had more tumors with poor prognostic features.

Rosenberg et al. (15,17,18) administered cyclophosphamide and adriamycin to a group of patients who were randomized to either amputation or conservative surgery plus radiation and compared the results in these patients with those in a group of historical controls treated at the National Cancer Institute by radical surgery alone. Both disease-free and overall survival were prolonged in patients receiving the adjuvant chemotherapy when compared with the historical controls. These data were the basis for a subsequent prospective, randomized trial to compare the use of adjuvant chemotherapy (adriamy-

172

cin, cyclophosphamide, and high-dose methotrexate with leucovorin rescue) with results in concomitant control patients not receiving adjuvant chemotherapy. Preliminary results of this trial appear to demonstrate a statistically significant improved disease-free survival in the chemotherapy patients (18), but final conclusions must await longer follow-up observations.

Although the foregoing studies suggest that adjuvant chemotherapy is effective in extending disease-free survival in patients with sarcomas, two other studies have not proved as promising. Edmonson et al. (3) compared 29 patients receiving chemotherapy (vincristine, cyclophosphamide, and dactinomycin alternated with vincristine, doxorubicin, and DTIC) with 31 patients undergoing surgery alone; patients were stratified according to primary site, tumor grade, and whether the sarcoma was being initially treated or was treated at the time of local recurrence. Preliminary results showed the time from treatment to the observation of metastases favored the adjuvant chemotherapy group, but this difference was not observed in patients with extremity tumors, and there was no difference in overall survival.

Lindberg et al. (9) reported preliminary results of an adjuvant chemotherapy trial which included patients with sarcoma equal to or greater than 5 cm in diameter and grades II or III histologically; patients were stratified according to histology, and all underwent conservative surgical resection combined with postoperative radiation therapy. The patients randomized to receive postoperative chemotherapy were administered vincristine, cyclophosphamide, adriamycin, and, after a total dose of 420 mg/m² of adriamycin, actinomycin D. Among 27 patients with chemotherapy, 9 developed distant metastases, but only 3 of the 20 control patients (no chemotherapy) developed metastases; this difference was not statistically significant. There were only 2 local recurrences observed, both in the control group, but both were salvaged by subsequent surgery. It is of interest that both groups in this small trial were compared with a historical control group; at 18 months the disease-free and overall survival was significantly better in both groups of the randomized study when compared with the historical controls. This difference was due to improved local control, possibly owing to refinements in radiotherapeutic technique, as the incidence of distant metastases was similar in the two time frames. These data further demonstrate the need for prospective, randomized trials and the pitfalls when comparisons are made with historical controls.

Several factors may account for Rosenberg's apparent demonstration of adjuvant chemotherapeutic efficacy while there was a lack of such efficacy in Edmonson's and Lindberg's trials. The chemotherapy employed differed in the various studies. The patient populations studied were probably different, and it is also possible that relatively small differences in dosage or timing may be important. Finally, the summarized results all represent preliminary observations that may change with time. It remains unclear whether any form of adjuvant chemotherapy will improve either disease-free or overall survival for adult patients with soft-tissue sarcomas.

Regional drug administration with (6,12,19) or without (4,5,14) complete vascular isolation of the extremity has been utilized for many years, but this method has not been studied in randomized trials. In isolation perfusion studies this approach has been utilized with the intent of improving local control, whereas continuous arterial infusion provides the possibility of an adjuvant therapy for both local and systemic tumor control.

Isolation perfusion for sarcomas has been performed using a variety of chemotherapeutic agents with and without hyperthermia and is obviously only applicable to patients with extremity sarcomas. It has the potential advantage of delivering high concentrations of drug to the primary tumor, much

173

higher than that achievable by systemic administration, and the prevention of escape of the chemotherapeutic agents into the systemic circulation, where they produce systemic effects. Hyperthermia may render sarcoma cells more susceptible to the chemotherapy administered and may actually kill tumor cells selectively over normal cells.

Regional perfusion alone has been reported to cause objective tumor regression (more than 50% decrease in size of measurable tumor) in 12 of 39 sarcoma patients, with minor responses in an additional 18 patients (6); a potential benefit is a more limited operation when regional perfusion is followed by delayed excision of the tumor, after response to chemotherapy. Nevertheless, five-year disease-free survival rates are similar to those obtained by surgery alone. Local recurrence rates of 17%–20% demonstrate no real advantage over either radical surgical excision or the combination of conservative surgery with radiation. In addition, the complications of regional perfusion include wound complications, thrombosis of arteries and veins, pulmonary emboli, cardiac arrhythmias, and bone marrow suppression; even experienced perfusionists report a number of deaths (6,12,19).

Preoperative arterial infusion therapy followed by radiation therapy prior to radical surgery and postoperative systemic chemotherapy has been reported for extremity sarcomas by Eilber et al. (4). With a median follow-up of 20 months, 2 of 65 patients demonstrated local recurrence; 4 patients required amputation because the sarcoma could not be removed with a lesser procedure despite this adjuvant therapy. The absolute survival appeared improved over that of a historical group of patients treated by resection alone. Unfortunately, this was not a randomized trial and similar results have been obtained using local treatment alone.

In addition to systemic postoperative chemotherapy, regional perfusion, and infusional therapy, systemic preoperative therapy has been used in conjunction with radiation therapy in an uncontrolled trial in an effort to decrease tumor size to make unresectable lesions resectable and to salvage limbs that might otherwise require amputation (10). Few patients have been treated in this manner and further investigation is required.

Conclusions

It seems probable that the combination of radiation therapy and conservative resection with histologically negative margins provides good local control of most soft-tissue sarcomas; however, whether or not there is an advantage to this combination over adequate soft-part resection remains unresolved. Similarly, the value of adjuvant chemotherapy remains unproven, although ongoing control trials may demonstrate its efficacy in a more convincing fashion. Perfusion therapy and infusion therapy may prove effective in decreasing local failure rates and in improving limb salvageability, but this has not yet been established.

References

1. Antman K, Blum R, Corson J, et al: Effective adjuvant chemotherapy for localized soft tissue sarcoma. Proc AACR 21:141, 1980.
2. das Gupta TK, Patel MK, Chaudhuri PK, Briele HA: The role of chemotherapy as an adjuvant to surgery in the initial treatment of primary soft tissue sarcomas in adults. J Surg Oncol 19:139–144, 1982.
3. Edmonson JH, Fleming TR, Ivins JC, et al: Reduced hematogenous metastasis in patients who receive systemic chemotherapy following excision of soft tissue

sarcomas: preliminary report. Proceedings of the American Association for Cancer Research 21:193, 1980.

4. Eilber FR, Mirra JJ, Grant TT, et al: Is amputation necessary for sarcomas?: A seven-year experience with limb salvage. Ann Surg 192:431–438, 1980.

5. Haskell CM, Silverstein MJ, Rangel DM, et al: Multimodality cancer therapy in man: a pilot study by arterial infusion. Cancer 33:1485–1490, 1974.

6. Krementz ET, Carter RD, Sutherland CM, Hutton I: Chemotherapy of sarcomas of the limbs by regional perfusion. Ann Surg 185:555–564, 1977.

7. Lindberg RD, Martin RG, Romsdahl MM: Surgery and postoperative radiotherapy in the treatment of soft tissue sarcomas in adults. Am J Roentgenol 123:123–129, 1975.

8. Lindberg RD, Martin RG, Romsdahl MM, Barkley HT: Conservative surgery and postoperative radiotherapy in 300 adults with soft-tissue sarcomas. Cancer 47:2391–2397, 1981.

9. Lindberg RD, Murphy WK, Benjamin RS, et al: Adjuvant chemotherapy in the treatment of primary soft tissue sarcomas: a preliminary report. *In* Management of Bone and Soft Tissue Tumors (The University of Texas MD Anderson Hospital and Tumor Institute, 21st Annual Clinical Conference on Cancer). Chicago, Year Book Medical Publishers, 1977, pp 343–352.

10. Lokich JJ: Preoperative chemotherapy in soft tissue sarcoma. Surg Gynecol Obstet 148:512–516, 1979.

11. Martin DS: The scientific basis for adjuvant chemotherapy. Cancer Treat Rev 8:169–189, 1981.

12. McBride CM: Regional chemotherapy for soft tissue sarcomas. *In* Management of Bone and Soft Tissue Tumors (The University of Texas MD Anderson Hospital and Tumor Institute, 21st Annual Clinical Conference on Cancer). Chicago, Year Book Medical Publishers, 1977, pp 353–360.

13. McNeer GP, Cantin J, Chu F, Nickson JJ: Effectiveness of radiation therapy in the management of sarcoma of the soft somatic tissues. Cancer 22:391–397, 1968.

14. Morton DL, Eilber FR, Townsend CM, et al: Limb salvage from a multidisciplinary treatment approach for skeletal and soft tissue sarcomas of the extremity. Ann Surg 184:268–278, 1976.

15. Rosenberg SA: Treatment of soft tissue sarcomas. *In* Surgical Oncology Research Workshop (September 9, 1981), pp 77–80, NIH Publ No 82-2444.

16. Rosenberg SA, Glatstein EJ: Perspectives on the role of surgery and radiation therapy in the treatment of soft tissue sarcomas of the extremities. Semin Oncol 8:190–200, 1981.

17. Rosenberg SA, Kent H, Costa J, Webber BI, Young R, Chabner B, Baker AR, Brennan MF, Chretien PB, Cohen MH, DeMoss EV, Sears HF, Seipp C, Simon R: Prospective randomized evaluation of the role of limb-sparing surgery, radiation therapy, and adjuvant chemoimmunotherapy in the treatment of adult soft-tissue sarcomas. Surgery 84:62–69, 1978.

18. Rosenberg SA, Tepper J, Glatstein E, Costa J, Baker A, Brennan M, DeMoss EV, Seipp C, Sindelar WF, Sugarbaker P, Wesley R: The treatment of soft-tissue sarcomas of the extremities: prospective randomized evaluations of (1) limb-sparing surgery plus radiation therapy compared with amputation and (2) the role of adjuvant chemotherapy. Ann Surg 196:305–315, 1982.

19. Stehlin JS, de Ipolyi PD, Giovanella BC, Gutierrez AE, Anderson RF: Soft tissue sarcomas of the extremity: multidisciplinary therapy employing hyperthermic perfusion. Am J Surg 130:643–646, 1975.

20. Suit HD, Proppe KH, Mankin HJ, Wood WC: Preoperative radiation therapy for sarcoma of soft tissue. Cancer 47:2269–2274, 1981.

21. Suit HD, Russell WO: Soft part tumors. Cancer 39:830–836, 1977.

22. Suit HD, Russell WO, Martin RG: Sarcoma of soft tissue: clinical and histopathologic parameters and response to treatment. Cancer 35:1478–1483, 1975.

23. Suit HD, Russell WO, Martin RG: Management of patients with sarcoma of soft tissue in an extremity. Cancer 21:1247–1255, 1973.

12 Management of Recurrent and Metastatic Sarcoma

Even following optimal local therapy of soft-tissue sarcomas, about half of all patients will experience treatment failure and ultimately succumb. The recurrence may be local/regional or at distant metastatic sites, but either problem will often require a therapeutic effort to achieve patient comfort. These patterns of treatment failure will be addressed individually.

Local Treatment Failure

Local recurrence must be considered the result of inadequate local therapy, and the frequency of this problem can be reduced by following the surgical principles outlined in Chapter 3. However, complete adherence to the surgical principle of "radical" resection with generous soft-tissue margins is not always feasible, particularly for anatomic sites such as the head and neck or retroperitoneum, and local treatment failure is more frequent under such circumstances. Compromise of the surgical margins may be on anatomic grounds (e.g., retroperitoneal sites or proximity to vital structures) or for the purpose of limb salvage, and this compromise may be an indication for postoperative radiation, as described in Chapter 11. Even patients requiring amputation of an extremity may have a less than optimal surgical margin in some instances, although local treatment failure occurs less frequently following these ablative procedures.

The clinical presentation of local recurrence is almost always that of a nodule or multiple nodules in the field of the prior operative resection. Recurrent disease manifested by regional lymph node involvement is an uncommon presentation with adult sarcoma patients, as noted in Chapter 1.

Distant Treatment Failure

Pulmonary metastases are the most frequent manifestation of distant recurrence after treatment of soft-tissue sarcomas. Although lung metastases are multiple in most patients with this problem, approximately 10% of patients with pulmonary metastases have a solitary lesion. Late in the course of the disease, pulmonary metastases are often accompanied by metastases at other sites, including the liver, the central nervous system, and even bone metastases.

The liver is an uncommon initial site of metastasis from soft-tissue sarcomas of the extremity or trunk. Visceral soft-tissue sarcomas may, however, metastasize to the liver primarily due to their relationship to the portal circulation. In addition, sarcomas arising from bone seem to have an increased incidence of hepatic metastases. It is, however, more common for hepatic metastases to develop when there is diffuse metastatic disease as previously noted.

Surgical Treatment

Local Recurrence

Treatment of local recurrences is usually dependent upon the type of initial treatment of the sarcoma. If the local recurrence follows an initial limited excision, the general principles described for operative treatment of primary soft-tissue sarcomas (Chapter 3) might still be applicable. First, such patients should be investigated for the possible presence of metastatic disease, which is more frequent when a sarcoma is locally recurrent. This work-up should be similar to the initial work-up advised for primary soft-tissue sarcomas (Chapter 2). In the absence of metastatic disease, if the sarcoma does not involve adjacent vital structures and can be resected with an envelope of normal tissue, it is reasonable to attempt a wide soft-tissue resection as if this were the initial treatment. If, however, vital structures are involved or there is a local recurrence following a wide soft-tissue resection or distal amputation, the patient should be considered for amputation. For thigh lesions, this would entail a hemipelvectomy; for upper arm lesions, an interscapulothoracic amputation would be required. It is important while performing such secondary surgery to resect the entire operative field of the previous operation, since this area is considered at risk for tumor cell implantation. Local recurrences following resection of primary trunk, abdominal wall, head and neck, or retroperitoneal sarcomas are difficult therapeutic problems; when possible, re-resection (with or without radiation therapy) is often useful palliative therapy and may prolong useful life.

Although it seems apparent that operation for local recurrence will not result in long-term disease-free survival as often as following the primary treatment, the results may be surprisingly good. Local recurrence rates are higher after reoperation, but overall long-term survival following reoperation may be 50% to 60% in these patients (17). These results may be due to the exclusion of patients with metastatic disease from reoperation, thereby selecting a reasonably favorable group of patients for re-resection.

Pulmonary Metastases

A surgical approach for pulmonary metastases has been employed for many years. Because sarcomas tend to metastasize hematogenously, pulmonary nodules may be the only detectable site of metastatic disease. Although about 90% of sarcoma patients with pulmonary metastases have multiple nodules, many such patients may benefit from an aggressive operative approach, almost as frequently as patients presenting with a solitary nodule. The results depend on the feasibility of total excision of all detectable metastatic disease.

Pulmonary metastases are usually first detected on a routine chest roentgenograph at some time following a "curative" resection. Symptoms do not usually occur until late in the clinical course; this is because pulmonary metastases are usually located in peripheral lung fields and, therefore, do not impinge on the bronchial tree until they are very large. This is in contrast to the clinical presentation of primary lung cancer, which is more commonly central, is often associated with early symptoms, and is usually detected because pulmonary symptoms have brought the patient to a physician.

When a pulmonary mass has been detected, further work-up is indicated before proceeding with treatment. A complete history may point to other sites of metastatic disease; physical examination may demonstrate local or, less commonly, lymph node recurrence. Routine blood chemistry values may show liver function abnormalities, which would suggest the need for further evaluation, possibly including liver scan, sonogram, or computed tomographic

Table 12-1.   Tomographic Findings in Patients with Metastatic Sarcoma on Chest X-Ray (33)

	Tomography			
	Solitary	Multiple	Unilateral	Bilateral
Chest x-ray: solitary	14	16		
unilateral			22	10

scan. In general, however, the routine use of scans or contrast studies is not indicated (see Chapter 2).

Chest x-ray alone should not be considered adequate evaluation of the pulmonary parenchyma in patients with sarcomas. Whole-lung tomography has proven very effective in delineating the full extent of disease (33). Patients who have solitary nodules on chest x-ray often will be found to have multiple nodules on tomograms; furthermore, and possibly more significantly, about one-third of patients whose tumor appears localized to one lung will be found to have bilateral nodules on tomograms (Table 12-1).

The recent use of computed tomography has led to investigation of this modality as a possibly more sensitive technique than whole-lung tomography. The usual method of tomography, with slices being performed at 1 cm cuts, will detect nodules of about 4 mm in size, whereas computed tomographic cuts will detect 2 to 3 mm nodules. However, in adults these additional lesions detected by computed tomography are frequently subpleural lymph nodes or small calcified granulomas (11), which limits the specificity of this test when compared with whole-lung tomography (Chapter 2). Later generation scanners may provide improved specificity to accompany this increased sensitivity of computed tomographic scanners over routine whole-lung tomography.

Contraindications to pulmonary resection for metastasis include severe, coexisting medical disease (such as severe chronic obstructive pulmonary disease), other sites of metastases, and massive bilateral pulmonary metastases. Percutaneous needle biopsy confirmation of diagnosis is not generally advisable unless operation is not to be performed and a tissue diagnosis is required before nonoperative therapy; it has the definite risks of pneumothorax and hemothorax and the potential risk of seeding sarcoma cells along the needle tract. In addition, even a percutaneous biopsy that is negative for cancer will not preclude an operation, owing to the possibility of a false-negative result.

Although the initial staging for primary lung cancer patients often includes bronchoscopy, cytology, mediastinoscopy, and on occasion scalene lymph node biopsy, these tests have not been useful for assessment of metastatic sarcomas. Since lung metastases are usually peripheral and subpleural, they do not shed cells into the tracheobronchial tree. In addition, although "metastases from metastases" have been described experimentally, and may occur clinically, it is uncommon to have hilar node metastases from metastatic sarcoma in the lung.

The operative technique for pulmonary metastasectomy is illustrated next. In general, wedge resection with conservation of as much lung tissue as possible is preferred to lobectomy or pneumonectomy. The subsequent incidence of local recurrence in the chest is low, and the possibility of future thoracotomies for other pulmonary sites of metastases certainly exists. Lobectomy or pneumonectomy should be reserved for the patient with massive disease that is not amenable to wedge resection or for the patient whose tumor is adherent to bronchus, major artery or vein.

Technique of Pulmonary Metastasectomy

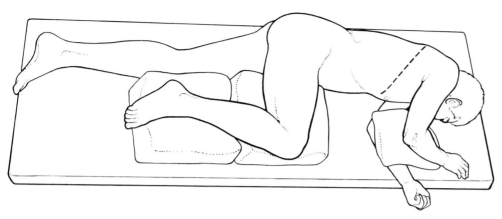

FIG. 12-1. The patient is prepared for a posterolateral thoracotomy. If possible, a Carlen's endotracheal tube should be introduced; when the lung is deflated, smaller lesions can be palpated than in an inflated lung. An adequate incision is necessary to carefully inspect and palpate the entire lung, even though preoperative roentgenographic studies may demonstrate only one mass.

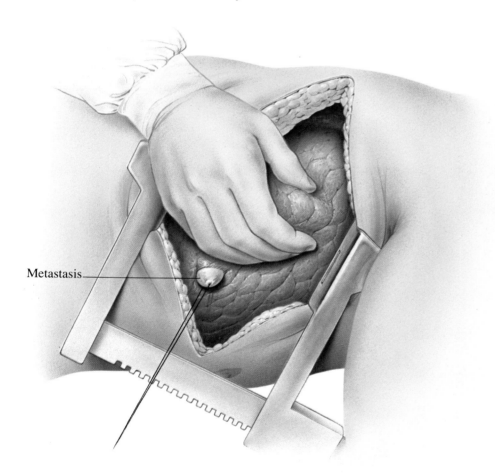

Metastasis

FIG. 12-2. The fifth or sixth interspace is entered and a Finochietto retractor introduced; it is rarely necessary to resect a rib for adequate exposure. Both the surgeon and the assistant should carefully palpate the entire pulmonary parenchyma, as well as the mediastinal lymph nodes, before resection is performed. All palpated lesions are marked with a suture; resection may distort the lung and make identification of previously noted lesions difficult without this technique.

179

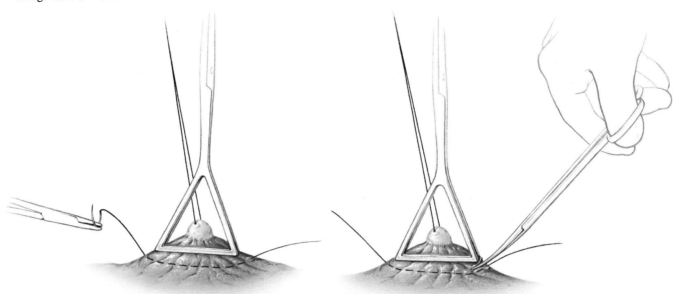

FIG. 12-3.   Most metastatic lesions are in a subpleural location; they tend to grow in an expansile fashion rather than infiltrating surrounding normal tissue. Accordingly, excision should involve resection of as small an amount of normal parenchyma as possible. Although this may be performed with a stapling device, postoperative computed tomography may not be reliable due to x-ray scatter produced by the staples. The mass is grasped with a lung clamp, the lung clamped around the lesion, and excision performed with a scalpel.

FIG. 12-4.   Following excision, the pulmonary parenchyma is reapproximated with a running 3-0 chromic suture. After all lesions have been excised, the lung is reinflated to check for air leaks. Massive metastatic lesions or lesions located centrally in a lobe may require lobectomy or pneumonectomy. Tumor adherent to the chest wall should be excised by chest wall resection and replacement with Marlex mesh or autogenous fascia.

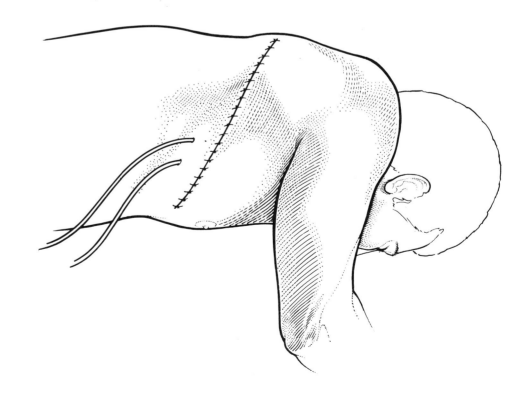

FIG. 12-5.   Following reexpansion of the lung, chest tubes are placed anteriorly and posteriorly and brought out inferior to the skin incision in the midaxillary line. The chest wall is closed in layers. Postoperative management of the chest tubes is identical with that employed after a thoracotomy for any other reason.

180

Table 12-2. Lung Resection for Metastatic Sarcoma

Institution		No. of patients	% 5-year survival	Median survival (mos)
UCLA* (22)	(b + st)	38	40	33
Minnesota (30)	(b + st)	42	36	?
Mayo Clinic (14)		112	29	18
RPMI (21)	(b + st)	50	~30	22
MGH (47)	(b + st)	21	21	?
MSKCC (29)	(b + st)	202	~25	?
NIH (33)	(b + st)	27	32	18

UCLA = University of California, Los Angeles; RPMI = Roswell Park Memorial Institute; MGH = Massachusetts General Hospital; MSKCC = Memorial Sloan-Kettering Cancer Center; NIH = National Institutes of Health.
* Adjuvant chemotherapy (Four-year survival in this report only)
b = bone sarcomas
st = soft-tissue sarcomas

Resection of pulmonary metastases from primary soft-tissue sarcomas has been employed for many years; surgeons from many different institutions have reported similar survival data following resection alone (14,21,22,29, 30,33,47). As yet, no improvement in survival with the addition of postoperative chemotherapy has been reported. Several prognostic variables may influence survival following resection (to be discussed).

Most series report that about 30% of patients undergoing resection of all pulmonary metastases will survive five years (Table 12-2). In general, this does not appear to differ according to histologic type, although the largest series, from Memorial Sloan-Kettering Cancer Center (29), does show some differences: five-year survival was 29% for synovial sarcoma, 27% for leiomyosarcoma, 21% for fibrosarcoma, but only 18% for neurofibrosarcoma. Data concerning number of nodules resected, number of thoracotomies, disease-free survival, tumor doubling time, and unilateral or bilateral disease were not presented. Osteosarcomas do not appear to have a different survival experience following resection of pulmonary metastases than soft-tissue sarcomas, and many authors group these tumors when reporting their results.

Various prognostic features have been examined in patients undergoing resection in an attempt to select those patients who will be most likely to benefit from resection of pulmonary metastases and those who will be most unlikely to benefit. The most important factor may be the thoroughness of the preoperative evaluation; among patients having unilateral nodules on a plain chest radiograph, about 30% will have bilateral disease on tomography (33). Patients who have a solitary nodule resected may have a somewhat better prognosis than patients with multiple nodules (33), but at least one large series has reported no statistically significant difference (46). The disease-free survival interval following initial treatment of the sarcoma may be an important prognostic factor; patients who have their metastasis detected more than two years following resection of the primary tumor (and thus, by inference, have a more slowly growing tumor) have an improved prognosis after resection than patients whose metastasis is detected and resected within two years of treatment of the primary tumor. The doubling time of the pulmonary metastasis was reported to be an important prognostic factor by Joseph et al. (23); they showed that all patients with doubling times of less than 20 days died of their tumor, but patients with doubling times of greater than 40 days did well (31). However, we have noted that metastases within the

181

same patient may have different growth rates (as determined from serial chest radiographs) and feel that thoracotomy should not be precluded on the basis of doubling time alone.

If patients develop new pulmonary metastases following pulmonary resection, the same principles previously elaborated should apply. Patients undergoing six to eight thoracotomies have been reported, with prolonged survivals.

Radiation Therapy

Soft-tissue sarcomas are responsive to radiation therapy, as described in Chapter 11. Although a less effective modality for initial management of the primary lesion than operative resection, radiation may be employed to palliate patients with local recurrence who are not amenable to secondary operative procedures. The results of therapy in this setting are not as striking as with previously untreated sarcomas, where approximately one-third of the lesions will achieve a complete clinical response. Nevertheless, it is a treatment method that should be considered for the palliation of selected patients with recurrent sarcomas.

Chemotherapy

Systemic chemotherapy may be utilized for patients with recurrence or metastases that are unsuitable for surgical resection. Regional chemotherapy has also been utilized for palliative treatment of selected patients with recurrent disease, but most patients anatomically suitable for this approach may be better managed by amputation. There was no really effective chemotherapeutic agent for adult sarcomas until the 1970s when the value of adriamycin was established (1,2,18). Many other drugs have been tried, with varying degrees of efficacy, and combination chemotherapy has been shown to be an effective approach in more recent years.

Adriamycin is one of the most effective single agents used in the management of metastatic soft-tissue sarcomas (Table 12-3). The literature review by Gottlieb et al. (18) demonstrated a 27% objective response rate to adriamycin; however, the median survival in the responders was only 8 months, a figure not statistically significantly different from the median survival in nonresponders (4 months). When response rates were correlated with the histologic appearance of the tumor, there were no significant differences among the various histologic types of soft-tissue sarcoma. The most important feature

Table 12-3.   Response Rates of Metastatic Soft-Tissue Sarcomas to Single-Agent Chemotherapy

Drug	% Response (complete + partial)
Adriamycin (18)	27
DTIC (3,20,26)	15
Methotrexate (44)	35
Cycloleucine (39)	7
High-dose methotrexate (24)	5
AMSA (43,51)	3
Vindesine (42)	3
cis-Platinum (7,9)	0
Chlorozotocin (32,41)	0
Piperazinedione (35)	0
Pyrazofurin (12)	0
Gallium nitrate (38)	0

regarding adriamycin administration appears to be related to dose: higher doses appear to correlate with higher response rates (34), but data demonstrating an effect on survival are meager. Thus, although objective responses are observed in a significant number of patients with metastatic soft-tissue sarcomas receiving adriamycin, the use of adriamycin alone does not appear to improve survival statistics.

DTIC (dacarbazine; dimethyltriazenoimidazole carboxamide) has been investigated in many series as a single agent (3,20,26); its main value, however, is in combination regimens (discussed later). The response rate to DTIC is about 15%; there appears to be minimal difference in effect by histologic type, but the numbers of patients are small. Survival data are also scarce.

Methotrexate was first reported in a large series of sarcoma patients in 1967 (48); the drug was administered intravenously, orally and/or intraarterially, thus making analysis difficult. In addition, the author did not define the response criteria employed. Of the 25 evaluable patients, 13 had "remissions" and 8 (32%) had complete responses which lasted from 2 to 45 months. A second series of 41 patients was more recently reported (44) which used standard response criteria similar to those of the cooperative chemotherapy groups: 15 patients (36%) had an objective response and 6 had a complete response. Partial responders had no improvement in survival time when compared with nonresponders, but complete responders lived significantly longer than the others. The response rate was 57% in patients with localized, unresectable sarcoma (including 5 of the 6 complete responders), but was only 26% in patients with metastatic disease. This study was part of a retrospective analysis which suggested that methotrexate alone was as effective as the combination of cyclophosphamide, vincristine, actinomycin D, and high-dose methotrexate or the combination of adriamycin, DTIC, and high-dose methotrexate. Exact comparisons between the patient groups are impossible from the published reports, and methotrexate has yet to be compared with aggressive combination chemotherapy in a randomized, prospective trial.

High-dose methotrexate was administered to 22 previously treated patients with metastatic soft-tissue sarcomas at the Roswell Park Memorial Institute (24); among 18 patients with evaluable tumors, only 1 responded. The authors suggested that methotrexate alone was of limited value when given as secondary chemotherapy. The lower response rate of methotrexate in this study may have been due to the previous treatment; methotrexate certainly appears to be an active drug and may be as effective as adriamycin as first-line chemotherapy, although they have not been directly compared.

Many other drugs that have been administered to patients with metastatic sarcomas appear to be relatively inactive. These include piperazinedione (35), chlorozotocin (32,41), vindesine (42), AMSA (43,51), cycloleucine (39), methyl-CCNU (15), pyrazofurin (12), dibromodulcitol (6), ICRF 159 (6), maytansine (6), gallium nitrate (38), and cis-platinum (7,9). These agents all have very low (0 to 7%) response rates in patients with previous treatment. An exception may be cis-platinum, which has been administered to a group of patients with "inoperable," previously untreated sarcoma, via intraarterial infusion, with objective responses noted in both bone and soft-tissue sarcomas (28). These results have yet to be confirmed in large numbers of patients with soft-tissue sarcomas or in patients with metastatic sarcoma.

Several drugs are often thought to have high response rates in patients with metastatic sarcomas, including vincristine, cyclophosphamide, and actinomycin D. Unfortunately, most reports include both children and adults; when these data were analyzed according to age, few adults responded to these drugs, but they are very active in children (34). This demonstrates one of

Table 12-4. Chemotherapeutic Regimens for Metastatic Sarcomas

Regimen	Response rate (%)
VCR, ACT D, CYC, ADR, MTX (10)	13.5
CYC, ADR, PLAT (12)	25
ADR, CYC/ACT D, DTIC (16)	20
ADR, CYC, MTX/ACT D, DTIC, VCR (36)	20
ACT D, meCCNU (50)	0
ADR, CYC, DTIC (5)	56
ADR, meCCNU (37)	45
ADR, ACT D (8)	28
ADR, VCR, MTX (25)	21
ADR, CYC, DTIC, ACT D (13)	21
ADR, DTIC, VCR, MTX/ADR, VCR, CYC, DTIC (27)	25

the differences between childhood and adult sarcomas that is not understood (Chapter 13).

The data previously discussed for single agents suggest that adriamycin, DTIC, and methotrexate are the most active single agents in the management of adult soft-tissue sarcomas. Most combination regimens have utilized one or more of these drugs, often with one or more of the less effective drugs: cyclophosphamide, vincristine, or actinomycin D. Such regimens have used the data obtained with childhood rhabdomyosarcoma as their rationale (Chapter 13). These regimens do, however, violate one of the tenets of combination chemotherapy: that all agents used in the combination should be active as single agents. Some of the results of using these combinations may reflect this.

Most effective chemotherapeutic regimens for adult sarcomas utilize adriamycin as one of the agents. The initial combination employed was adriamycin plus DTIC (19), a regimen combining two of the active single agents. The observed response rate, 41%, was higher than that seen with either agent in previous series. Neither the tumor histology nor the sites of metastases appeared to affect the response rate. A later report (18) showed that patients who responded had a statistically significantly improved survival when compared with nonresponders or with patients treated by adriamycin alone in the previous trial. Thus, this combination appeared effective in increasing both response rate and survival in patients with metastatic sarcomas.

Later studies have added vincristine (18) and/or cyclophosphamide (5) to the combination of adriamycin and DTIC. Neither vincristine added alone nor cyclophosphamide added alone appeared to significantly improve the results obtained with adriamycin and DTIC (4). When both cyclophosphamide and vincristine were added to adriamycin and DTIC, the response rate was slightly higher (50%) than with the historical series of adriamycin plus DTIC, but neither response duration nor survival was improved (49). A recent review also suggests that combining vincristine and/or actinomycin D with adriamycin and DTIC offers no advantage over the two-drug regimen (45); this is a not unexpected finding because neither vincristine nor actinomycin D has documented efficacy in metastatic adult sarcomas.

Numerous other combination chemotherapy regimens have been evaluated in patients with metastatic soft-tissue sarcomas, but few randomized trials have been attempted. In addition, most other regimens have included drugs that are inactive as single agents. The partial listing of combination chemotherapy regimens in Table 12-4 reflects the lower response rates seen with these drugs when compared with adriamycin and DTIC.

The current status of chemotherapy for sarcomas suggests: 1) Adriamycin, DTIC, and methotrexate are the most active single agents, but the survival of responders when compared with nonresponders is not prolonged. 2) Adults respond much less favorably and to different drugs than do children. 3) The most active combination in adult sarcomas appears to be adriamycin and DTIC; the addition of other agents has yet to show an advantage. 4) Responders to adriamycin plus DTIC have an improved survival when compared with nonresponders, or even with patients who respond to adriamycin alone or DTIC alone. 5) Response is not predicted by histology, primary site, or site of the sarcoma metastases.

References

1. Benjamin RS, Baker LH, Rodriguez V, Moon TE, O'Bryan RM, Stephens RL, Sinkovics JG, Thigpen T, Kind GW, Bottomley R, Groppe CW, Bodey GP, Gottlieb JA: The chemotherapy of soft tissue sarcomas in adults. *In* Management of Primary Bone and Soft Tissue Tumors. Chicago, Year Book Medical Publishers, 1977, pp 309–316.
2. Benjamin RS, Wiernik PH, Bachur NR: Adriamycin: a new effective agent in the therapy of disseminated sarcomas. Med Pediatr Oncol 1:63–76, 1975.
3. Beretta G, Bonadonna G, Bajetta E, Tancini G, DeLena M, Azzarelli A, Veronesi U: Combination chemotherapy with DTIC (NSC-45388) in advanced malignant melanoma, soft tissue sarcomas, and Hodgkin's disease. Cancer Treat Rep 60:205–211, 1976.
4. Beretta G, Fraschini P, Tedeschi L: Chemotherapy of soft tissue sarcomas. Oncology 37(Suppl 1):92–96, 1980.
5. Blum RH, Corson JM, Wilson RE, Greenberger JS, Canellos GP, Frei E: Successful treatment of metastatic sarcomas with cyclophosphamide, adriamycin, and DTIC (CAD). Cancer 46:1722–1726, 1980.
6. Borden E, Ash A, Rosenbaum C, Lerner H: Phase II evaluation of dibromodulcitol (DBD), ICRF 159, and maytansine for sarcomas. Am J Clin Oncol 5:417–420, 1982.
7. Bramwell VHC, Brugasolas A, Mouridsen HT, Cheix F, DeJager R, van Oosterom AT, Vendrik CP, Pinedo HM, Sylvester R, DePauw M: E.O.R.T.C. phase II study of cisplatin in cyvadic-resistant soft tissue sarcoma. Eur J Cancer 15:1511–1513, 1979.
8. Brenner DE, Chang P, Wiernik PH: Doxorubicin and dactinomycin therapy for advanced sarcomas. Cancer Treat Rep 65:231–236, 1981.
9. Brenner J, Magill GB, Sordillo PP, Chang EW, Yagoda A: Phase II trial of cisplatin (CPDD) in previously treated patients with advanced sarcoma. Cancer 50:2031–2033, 1982.
10. Bryant BM, Wiltshaw E: Results of the Royal Marsden Hospital second soft tissue sarcoma schedule (STS II) chemotherapy regimen in the management of advanced sarcomas. Cancer Treat Rep 64:689–692, 1980.
11. Chang AE, Schaner EG, Conkle DM, Flye MW, Doppman JL, Rosenberg SA: Evaluation of computed tomography in the detection of pulmonary metastases: a prospective study. Cancer 43:913–916, 1979.
12. Cormier WJ, Hahn RG, Edmonson JH, Eagan RT: Phase II study in advanced sarcoma: randomized trial of pyrazofurin versus combination cyclophosphamide, doxorubicin, and *cis*-dichlordiamminplatinum (II) (CAP). Cancer Treat Rep 64:655–658, 1980.
13. Creagan ET, Edmonson JH, Hahn RG, Ahmann DL, Bisel HF, Eagan RT: A preliminary study of cyclophosphamide (NSC-26271), adriamycin (NSC-123127), imidazole carboxamide (NSC-45388), and actinomycin D (NSC-3053) with or without MER-BCG in patients with advanced sarcomas. Med Pediatr Oncol 4:85–86, 1978.

14. Creagan ET, Fleming TR, Edmonson JH, Pairolero PC: Pulmonary resection for metastatic non-osteogenic sarcoma. Cancer 44:1908–1912, 1979.

15. Creagan ET, Hahn RG, Ahmann DL, Edmonson JH, Bisel HF, Eagan RT: A comparative clinical trial evaluating the combination of adriamycin, DTIC, and vincristine, the combination of actinomycin D, cyclophosphamide, and vincristine, and a single agent, methyl-CCNU, in advanced sarcomas. Cancer Treat Rep 30:1385–1387, 1976.

16. Dalley DN, Levi JA, Nesbitt RA, Tattersall MHN, Woods RL, Fox RM, Aroney RS: Cyclical combination chemotherapeutic regimen in adult soft tissue sarcoma. Cancer Clin Trials 4:163–165, 1981.

17. Giuliano AE, Eilber FR, Morton DL: The management of locally recurrent soft-tissue sarcoma. Ann Surg 196:87–91, 1982.

18. Gottlieb JA, Baker LH, O'Brien RM, Sinkovics JG, Hoogstraten B, Quagliana JM, Rivkin SE, Bodey GP, Rodriguez VT, Blumenschein GR, Saiki JH, Coltman C, Burgess MA, Sullivan P, Thigpen T, Bottomley R, Bakerzak S, Moon TE: Adriamycin (NSC-123127) used alone and in combination for soft tissue and bony sarcomas. Cancer Chemother Rep 6:271–282, 1975.

19. Gottlieb JA, Baker LH, Quagliana JM, Luce JK, Whitecar JP, Sinkovics JG, Rivkin SE, Brownlee R, Frei E: Chemotherapy of sarcomas with a combination of adriamycin and dimethyl triazeno imidazole carboxamide. Cancer 30:1632–1638, 1972.

20. Gottlieb JA, Benjamin RS, Baker LH, O'Bryan RM, Sinkovics JG, Hoogstraten B, Quagliana JM, Rivkin SE, Bodey GP, Rodriguez V, Blumenschein GR, Saiki JH, Coltman C, Burgess MA, Sullivan P, Thigpen T, Bottomley R, Balcerzak S, Moon TE: Role of DTIC (NSC-45388) in the chemotherapy of sarcomas. Cancer Treat Rep 60:199–203, 1976.

21. Huang MN, Edgerton F, Takita H, Douglass HO, Karakousis C: Lung resection for metastatic sarcoma. Am J Surg 135:804–806, 1978.

22. Huth JF, Holmes EC, Vernon SE, Callery CD, Ramming KP, Morton DL: Pulmonary resection for metastatic sarcoma. Am J Surg 140:9–16, 1980.

23. Joseph WL, Morton DL, Adkins PC: Variation in tumor doubling time in patients with pulmonary metastatic disease. J Surg Oncol 3:143–149, 1971.

24. Karakousis CP, Rao U, Carlson M: High-dose methotrexate as secondary chemotherapy in metastatic soft-tissue sarcomas. Cancer 46:1345–1348, 1980.

25. Kaufman JH, Catane R, Douglass HO: Combined adriamycin, vincristine, and methotrexate in advanced, adult, soft-tissue sarcoma. NY State J Med 77:742–743, 1977.

26. Luce JK, Thurman WG, Isaacs BL, Talley RW: Clinical trials with the antitumor agent 5-(3,3-dimethyl-1-triazeno) imidazole-4-carboxamide (NSC-45388). Cancer Chemother Rep 54:119–124, 1970.

27. Lynch G, Magill GB, Sordillo P, Golbey RB: Combination chemotherapy of advanced sarcomas in adults with "CYOMAD" (S7). Cancer 50:1724–1727, 1982.

28. Mavligit GM, Benjamin R, Patt YZ, Jaffe N, Chuang V, Wallace S, Murray J, Ayala A, Johnston S, Hersh EM, Calvo DB: Intra-arterial cis-platinum for patients with inoperable skeletal tumors. Cancer 48:1–4, 1981.

29. McCormack PM, Martini N: The changing role of surgery for pulmonary metastases. Ann Thorac Surg 28:139–145, 1979.

30. Morrow CE, Vassilopoulos PP, Grage TB: Surgical resection for metastatic neoplasms of the lung: experience at the University of Minnesota Hospitals. Cancer 45:2981–2985, 1980.

31. Morton DL, Joseph WL, Ketcham AS, Geelhoed GW, Adkins PC: Surgical resection and adjunctive immunotherapy for selected patients with multiple pulmonary metastases. Ann Surg 178:360–366, 1973.

32. Mouridsen HT, Bramwell VHC, Lacave J, Metz R, Vendrik C, Hild J, McCreanney J, Sylvester R: Treatment of advanced soft tissue sarcomas with chlorozotocin: a phase II trial of the EORTC soft tissue and bone sarcoma group. Cancer Treat Rep 65:509–511, 1981.

33. Neifeld JP, Michaelis LL, Doppman JL: Suspected pulmonary metastases: correla-

tion of chest x-ray, whole lung tomograms, and operative findings. Cancer 39:383–387, 1977.

34. Pinedo HM, Kenis Y: Chemotherapy of advanced soft tissue sarcomas in adults. Cancer Treat Rev 4:67–86, 1977.

35. Presant CA, Bartolucci AA: Phase II trial of piperazinedione in metastatic sarcoma. Am J Clin Oncol 5:185–187, 1982.

36. Presant CA, Lowenbraun S, Bartolucci AA, Smalley RV: Metastatic sarcomas: chemotherapy with adriamycin, cyclophosphamide and methotrexate alternating with actinomycin D, DTIC, and vincristine. Cancer 47:457–465, 1981.

37. Rivkin SE, Gottlieb JA, Thigpen T, el Mawla NG, Saiki J, Dixon DO: Methyl CCNU and adriamycin for patients with metastatic sarcomas: a Southwest Oncology Group Study. Cancer 46:446–451, 1980.

38. Saiki JH, Baker LH, Stephens RL, Fabian CJ, Kraut EH, Fletcher WS: Gallium nitrate in advanced soft tissue and bone sarcomas: a southwest oncology group study. Cancer Treat Rep 66:1673–1674, 1982.

39. Savlov ED, MacIntyre JM, Knight E, Wolter J: Comparison of doxorubicin with cycloleucine in the treatment of sarcomas. Cancer Treat Rep 65:21–27, 1981.

40. Schoenfeld DA, Rosenbaum C, Horton J, Wolter JM, Falkson G, DeConti RC: A comparison of adriamycin versus vincristine and adriamycin, and cyclophosphamide versus vincristine, actinomycin D, and cyclophosphamide for advanced sarcoma. Cancer 50:2757–2762, 1982.

41. Sordillo PP, Magill GB, Gralla RJ: Chlorozotocin: phase II evaluation in patients with advanced sarcomas. Cancer Treat Rep 65:513–514, 1981.

42. Sordillo PP, Magill GB, Gralla RJ: Phase II evaluation of vindesine sulfate in patients with advanced sarcomas. Cancer Treat Rep 65:515–516, 1981.

43. Sordillo PP, Magill GB, Gralla RJ, Golbey RB: Phase II evaluation of 4'-(9-acridinylamino)-methanesulfon-m-anisidide (AMSA) in patients with advanced sarcoma. Cancer Treat Rep 64:1129–1130, 1980.

44. Subramanian S, Wiltshaw E: Chemotherapy of sarcoma: a comparison of three regimens. Lancet 1:683–686, 1978.

45. Sutow WW, Maurer HM: Chemotherapy of sarcomas—a perspective. Semin Oncol 8:207–214, 1981.

46. Takita H, Edgerton F, Merrin C, Douglass HO, Karakousis C: Management of multiple lung metastases. J Surg Oncol 12:199–205, 1979.

47. Wilkins EW, Head JM, Burke JF: Pulmonary resection for metastatic neoplasms in the lung: experience at the Massachusetts General Hospital. Am J Surg 135:480–483, 1978.

48. Wiltshaw E: Methotrexate in treatment of sarcomata. Br Med J 2:142–145, 1967.

49. Yap B-S, Baker LH, Sinkovics JG, Rivkin SE, Bottomley R, Thigpen T, Burgess MA, Benjamin RS, Bodey GP: Cyclophosphamide, vincristine, adriamycin, and DTIC (CYVADIC) combination chemotherapy for the treatment of advanced sarcomas. Cancer Treat Rep 64:93–98, 1980.

50. Yap B-S, Benjamin RS, Burgess MA, Murphy WK, Sinkovics JG, Bodey GP: A phase II evaluation of methyl-CCNU and actinomycin D in the treatment of advanced sarcomas in adults. Cancer 47:2807–2809, 1981.

51. Yap B-S, Plager C, Benjamin RS, Murphy WK, Legha SS, Bodey GP: Phase II evaluation of AMSA in adult sarcomas. Cancer Treat Rep 65:341–343, 1981.

13 Special Aspects of Childhood Sarcomas

Soft-tissue sarcomas in infants and children are unusual tumors, representing the fourth most common malignant disease in patients under 15 years of age (Table 13-1) (42). They represent a significant percentage of the solid neoplasms arising in children and frequently present both diagnostic and therapeutic dilemmas. In recent years a great deal of interest has centered on the marked improvement in disease control that has resulted from combined-modality treatment of rhabdomyosarcomas. Other forms of soft-tissue sarcoma arising in childhood are much less common, less is known about their natural history, and combined-modality therapy trials for these lesions are nonexistent. This chapter will review the sarcomas arising in childhood and the differences when compared with adult sarcomas. The main thrust of this chapter will be the discussion of the emerging data on rhabdomyosarcomas.

All sarcomas described in children have also been reported in adults, but the histologic distribution differs markedly (16,30,34,35,38,41). In children the two most common sarcomas are rhabdomyosarcomas and fibrosarcomas (27), constituting over 60% of all sarcomas (Table 13-2). Other sarcomas are less common and, in a recent review (27), 15% were not able to have a specific histology determined. This distribution is in contrast to the distribution of sarcomas found in adults.

A recent review of 892 histologically diagnosed soft-tissue sarcomas in infants and children below the age of 19 was made from data of the End Results Section of the National Cancer Institute (27). All children were initially diagnosed between 1955 and 1971. The epidemiology of these tumors is of

Table 13-1. Frequency of Cancers in Children (42)

	Rate/million
Leukemia	42.1
CNS tumor	23.9
Lymphoma	13.2
Soft-tissue sarcoma	8.4
Neuroblastoma	7.9
Wilms' tumor	7.5
Bone tumors	5.6

Table 13-2. Frequency of Sarcomas in Childhood (27)

	No.	Male	Female
Rhabdomyosarcoma	385	227	158
Fibrosarcoma	182	112	70
Angiosarcoma	59	35	24
Synovial sarcoma	50	27	23
Leiomyosarcoma	29	9	20
Liposarcoma	26	11	15
Malignant schwannoma	25	14	11
Other	136	87	49
Total	892	522	370

interest and differed somewhat from the epidemiology of adult soft-tissue sarcomas. In children, about 90% of the sarcomas were present in whites compared with only 10% in blacks. This proportion, however, approximates the racial distributions of patients in the reporting hospitals.

The most common primary site of the soft-tissue sarcomas in childhood was the head and neck (Table 13-3), with extremities and trunk being less commonly the site of origin. The genitourinary tract was the primary site for 12% of the sarcomas, but the great majority of these were rhabdomyosarcomas (Table 13-4). This contrasts markedly with the site distribution noted in adults, where the extremities are the primary site for most sarcomas, and only liposarcomas and leiomyosarcomas are frequently found in the retroperitoneum. As can be seen in Table 13-4, other primary sites varied considerably depending upon the histology; although rhabdomyosarcomas most commonly originated in the head and neck or genitourinary tract, synovial sarcomas almost invariably were located in the extremities; most leiomyosarcomas originated in the gastrointestinal tract.

Males appeared to have a higher incidence of sarcomas than females, with 59% of the sarcomas being diagnosed in male patients (Table 13-2). Only leiomyosarcomas and liposarcomas had a female preponderance. The extent of disease at presentation was localized in 55%, regional in 20%, and disseminated in 25%. Again, however, this depended on the histology of the primary tumor (Table 13-5), as fibrosarcomas, liposarcomas, and leiomyosarcomas usually presented with localized disease, but rhabdomyosarcomas were frequently disseminated, although often not clinically apparent. These data correlated with the prognosis of the various histologic types.

Treatment of most childhood soft-tissue sarcomas involves a surgical approach despite the addition of other important modalities in recent years.

Table 13-3. Site of Pediatric Soft-Tissue Sarcomas (27)

Head and Neck	30%
Lower extremity	17%
Trunk	16%
Genitourinary	12%
Upper extremity	8%
Other	17%

Table 13-4. Site of Origin of Pediatric Soft-Tissue Sarcomas Correlated with Histology (27)

Histology	Site				
	H&N	Ext.	GU	Trunk	Other
Rhabdomyosarcoma	144	53	76	44	68
Fibrosarcoma	44	54	7	35	42
Angiosarcoma	17	10	1	14	17
Synovial sarcoma	1	40		1	8
Leiomyosarcoma	1	1	3	1	23
Liposarcoma	4	12		8	2
Malignant schwannoma	2	3	3	9	11

Table 13-5. Extent of Disease at Initial Presentation Correlated with Histology (27)

Histology	Localized (%)	Regional (%)	Disseminated (%)
Rhabdomyosarcoma	41	23	36
Angiosarcoma	57	19	24
Malignant schwannoma	58	29	13
Synovial sarcoma	62	19	19
Leiomyosarcoma	70	17	13
Liposarcoma	79	12	9
Fibrosarcoma	80	12	8

Similar principles to those described earlier (Chapter 3) for the treatment of adult soft-tissue sarcomas should, in general, be followed in the management of childhood soft-tissue sarcomas, but the important role of chemotherapy for childhood rhabdomyosarcoma does lead to a number of modifications. Although rhabdomyosarcoma appears to be a different entity in children, when compared with adults, most other histologic types of sarcoma appear to have a similar natural history. There are no combined-modality treatment protocols for childhood sarcomas other than rhabdomyosarcomas that have utilized radiation and/or chemotherapy with surgery. Most childhood sarcomas are too rare to ever expect a valid randomized prospective trial to establish the benefits of combined-modality therapy, so historical series will need to be used for future reference points.

Fibrosarcoma

Fibrosarcoma is the second most frequent sarcoma in patients below the age of 19. A few small series have been reported (3,6,7,9,11,36,37), and prognostic variables have not been well delineated. Within a group of 182 patients compiled over 16 years (26), there were 112 males and 70 females; 160 patients were white, and 22 were black. The primary sites included 19% in the trunk, 19% in the head and neck, 18% in the lower extremity, and 12% in the upper extremity (Fig. 13-1). Although many patients in the literature have been diagnosed within the first year of life (36), only 16% of the patients in this series were diagnosed in children below the age of 2 years. The overall survival in patients with fibrosarcomas approximated 80% at 5 years, a figure much superior to that noted for adult fibrosarcomas. The series reported from the Mayo Clinic (36) suggested that children less than 5 years of age had a local recurrence rate of 43%, but only a 7.3% chance of developing metastatic spread. They also suggested that children 10 or older had a metastatic rate of 50% at 5 years, a figure approximately that seen in adults. When our group of patients was evaluated (26), age did not correlate with survival. A factor that did correlate with survival was that of stage at diagnosis, as patients with localized disease had a far superior prognosis when compared with patients having regional or disseminated sarcoma.

The site of the primary tumor also correlated with survival. Patients with upper extremity lesions were almost invariably cured, probably owing to the small amount of surrounding soft tissue and, therefore, early detection of the lesion. Retroperitoneal fibrosarcomas, however, had a poor prognosis, with only about 15% of the patients having prolonged disease-free survival. This was likely due to late diagnosis with invasion of surrounding structures, making curative resection frequently impossible.

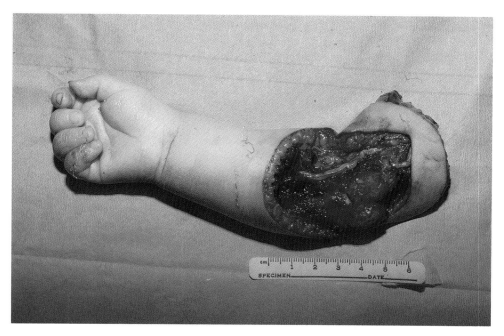

FIG. 13-1. Amputation specimen of fibrosarcoma in a one-year-old child that recurred after prior local resection.

Many benign variants of fibrosarcoma have been described in infants (3,4,7,19). The congenital fibrosarcomas are low-grade tumors, do not metastasize, but do tend to recur locally. Another group of tumors, with names including diffuse infantile fibromatosis, fibromatosis coli, dermal fibromatosis, fibrous hamartoma of infancy, cranial fasciitis of childhood, and congenital and aggressive infantile fibromatosis, probably resemble the dermatofibrosarcoma protuberans seen in adults (at least as far as the clinical behavior is concerned) and should be treated by a wide local excision with adequate margins. This should be accomplished without sacrificing significant function of the extremity and without amputation. It appears that this group of tumors will often be cured by this approach; local recurrences and distant metastases are extremely rare if local resection is adequate. The age-related prognosis for fibrosarcoma at the Mayo Clinic may, in part, be due to the inclusion of many of these benign variants in their series. At the time of recurrence, more aggressive surgical therapy is appropriate.

Little information is available regarding radiation therapy or chemotherapy in the management of childhood fibrosarcoma. Experience with a small series of cases treated at the Medical College of Virginia suggests that these tumors respond poorly, if at all, to chemotherapy. Patients developing pulmonary metastatic disease should be treated in a manner similar to that for adults, and if possible all metastatic disease in the lungs should be resected. Radiation therapy and/or chemotherapy should be attempted for other metastatic sites. Occasional long-term survivals may be expected with this approach.

Liposarcoma

Tumors of fat cell origin are rare in childhood and compose only about 3% of sarcomas in this age group. Only about 1% of liposarcomas occur in children (8). They tend to have a slight female predominance and are found most often in the extremities and trunk. Liposarcomas have better survival statistics in children than in adults, which may be due to the less common occurrence of liposarcoma in the retroperitoneal area in children than in adults. The disease-free survival rate with this primary site is 15%. In our recent series including all sites (27), the five-year survival was 70%. Treatment consists of adequate soft-part resection, with adjuvant radiotherapy when inadequate surgical margins have been obtained. The exact role of chemotherapy has not been established, but active agents include vincristine, actinomycin D, cyclophosphamide, adriamycin, and DTIC.

A very rare condition may occur in infants called lipoblastomatosis (2,17). This is a lobulated tumor composed of benign lipoblasts and may be confused with well-differentiated myxoid liposarcoma. Proper treatment of this entity is local excision.

Leiomyosarcoma

Smooth muscle tumors in children constitute approximately 2% to 3% of soft-tissue sarcomas in children; fewer than 5% of all leiomyosarcomas occur in children (10). Few series have discussed the incidence or site of these tumors. There appears to be a slight female to male predominance, and many are retroperitoneal (27). The problem with smooth muscle tumors continues to be the differential diagnosis of leiomyoma as opposed to leiomyosarcoma; this rests on the presence of metastatic disease and/or the number of mitoses per high-power field. Our review of 29 patients with leiomyosarcomas suggested an excellent survival rate (27), but the histologic slides were not reviewed to determine whether these were indeed all leiomyosarcomas or may have included leiomyomas. The Mayo Clinic series of 10 patients suggested survival rates as poor in childhood as in adults, with only 3 patients (of 10) with prolonged disease-free survivals (1). Treatment of these tumors continues to be adequate soft-part resection. Leiomyoma, the benign counterpart, requires only simple local excision, as in adults.

Synovial Sarcomas

Synovial sarcomas are rare in childhood, and compose only about 5% of childhood soft-tissue sarcomas (5,23,27,30). Only about 10% of all synovial sarcomas occur prior to the age of 16. They are evenly distributed between sexes, and most commonly originate in the distal portion of an extremity. Survival following surgery for these sarcomas in children is similar to that in adults, with 40% to 60% of patients remaining disease-free after primary surgical therapy. Results of treatment of recurrences, however, are poor. This suggests that these sarcomas must be treated aggressively at the time of initial operation to prevent the local recurrence which is so often fatal. With the relatively poor survival rates noted in some series, the best approach might be to treat these patients with combined-modality regimens. The combination of vincristine, actinomycin D, cyclophosphamide, adriamycin, and DTIC has produced regressions of synovial sarcomas.

Malignant Fibrous Histiocytoma

Although malignant fibrous histiocytoma is the most common soft-tissue sarcoma diagnosed in adults, few have been reported in children. We have treated six children with this tumor; all six underwent surgery, one had chemotherapy, and one had radiation therapy plus chemotherapy (after total surgical resection) (Fig. 13-2). All children remain free of tumor, two to six years later. This suggests that malignant fibrous histiocytomas may have a better prognosis in children than adults, but the number of patients is obviously small.

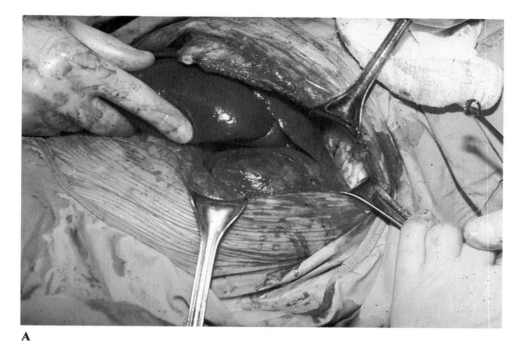

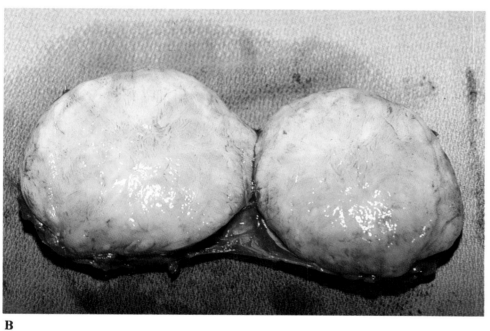

FIG. 13-2. Retroperitoneal malignant fibrous histiocytoma in a 15-year-old shown at time of operation (**A**). Total resection was accomplished and the surgical specimen is shown in **B**.

Rhabdomyosarcoma

Rhabdomyosarcoma represents between 5% and 15% of all malignant solid tumors in children under the age of 15 and is the most common soft-tissue sarcoma in this age group. Advances in our knowledge of the clinical presentation, pathology, and natural history of childhood rhabdomyosarcoma have been made by means of the national clinical trials of the Intergroup Rhabdomyosarcoma Study (IRS). These trials have addressed a number of therapeutic questions in the first two protocols (IRS I and II) and attempt to further refine therapy in IRS III.

193

Background of IRS Trials

Prior to the use of effective radiotherapy and the subsequent development of effective chemotherapy, surgical approaches were the only form of treatment for children with rhabdomyosarcoma, and most early reports described long-term survival in the range of 15% (24). Even those patients appearing to have clinically localized disease had only a 25% long-term survival following surgical resection (22). After 1965, it became clear that intensive radiotherapy (in the range of 5000–6000 rads over 5–6 weeks) did result in significant tumor regression in many instances, and local control was achieved in some patients by this means alone (29). The major subsequent improvement in prognosis for this disease can be attributed to the development of effective chemotherapy programs in the early 1960s, primarily the use of actinomycin D, vincristine, and cyclophosphamide. In retrospect, it is apparent that the majority of patients with rhabdomyosarcoma have distant metastatic disease at the time of initial diagnosis, whether clinically apparent or not, and systemic therapy must be considered a vital part of the overall treatment plan.

Effective drug combination treatment programs were reported in pilot trials of adjuvant therapy (18,31), but the major advance in the evaluation of this form of management was a prospective clinical trial carried out in 1967 by the Children's Cancer Study Group (CCSG) (15). This study compared patients receiving chemotherapy (vincristine, actinomycin D, and cyclophosphamide) following surgical resection with a group of patients treated by surgical resection without chemotherapy. This randomized trial clearly demonstrated that patients who had surgical resection (with or without microscopic residual tumor) *and* postoperative chemotherapy had survival rates superior to the concomitant controls. The important role of adjuvant combination chemotherapy for childhood rhabdomyosarcoma was established by this trial, and this led to the larger, more detailed national study begun in 1972, the IRS.

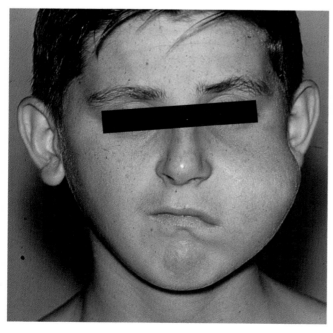

FIG. 13-3. Childhood rhabdomyosarcoma arising in the cheek and parotid region.

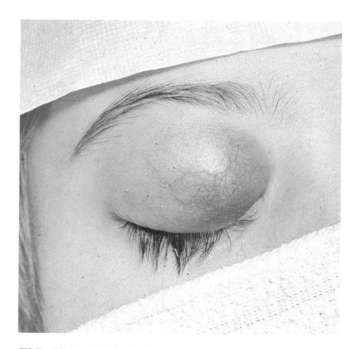

FIG. 13-4. Orbital rhabdomyosarcoma in child.

194

The primary objectives of the IRS were to refine the therapeutic program for patients who had resectable rhabdomyosarcomas, to establish effective treatment programs for lesions that either were not resectable or were metastatic, and to collect a group of patients that was large enough to permit better characterization of this disease. Data obtained in the IRS on the clinical presentation, pathology, and natural history of this disease demonstrated a number of features that are clearly different from those observed in adults with rhabdomyosarcoma or other soft-part sarcomas.

Clinical Features

Rhabdomyosarcomas in childhood have a different anatomic distribution than observed with soft-part sarcomas in adults. The head and neck area, including the orbit, was the most frequent site (38%) in the IRS, followed by the genitourinary tract (21%), extremities (18%), trunk and retroperitoneum (14%), and miscellaneous sites (9%) (25) (Figs. 13-3 through 13-7). This distribution affects both the clinical course of the disease and the treatment plan, and the prognosis observed in this study depended upon both the primary site and variations in histologic type of rhabdomyosarcoma (discussed later).

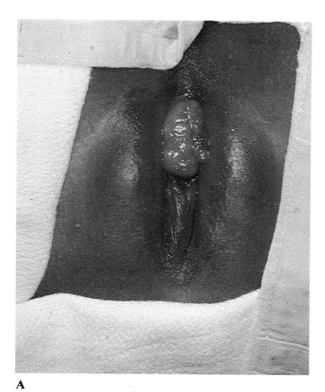

A

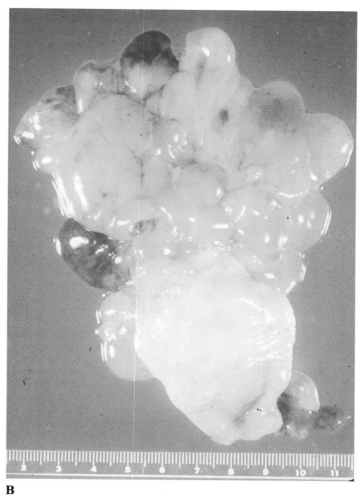

B

FIG. 13-5. Childhood rhabdomyosarcoma arising from vagina and presenting at introitus as classical sarcoma botryoides (A). Surgical specimen of a similar lesion is shown in B.

195

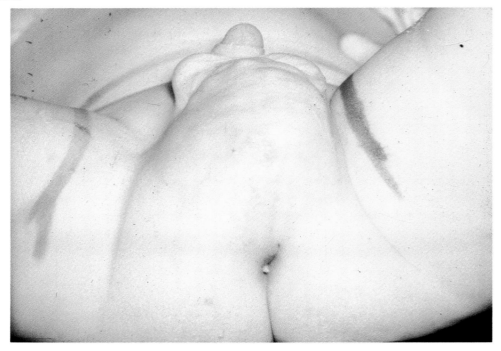

FIG. 13-6.   Childhood rhabdomyosarcoma arising from perineal site.

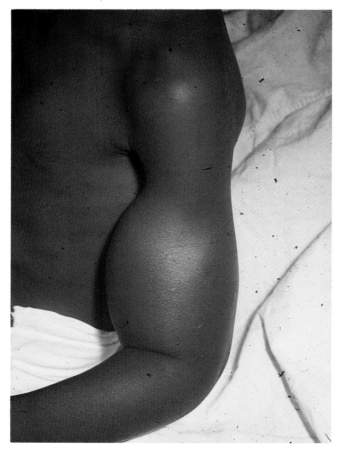

FIG. 13-7.   Rhabdomyosarcoma in upper extremity of a child.

Table 13-6. Postsurgical Staging Schema Utilized in IRS I and II

Group	Classification
I	Localized disease, completely resected (Microscopic confirmation of complete resection) A. Confined to organ or muscle of origin B. Infiltration outside organ or muscle of origin (still localized); no lymph node involvement
II	Regional disease, grossly resected A. Gross resection with microscopic residual demonstrated by involvement in the margin of resection; no lymph node involvement B. Gross resection of primary lesion associated with involved regional lymph nodes and/or extension into adjacent organ(s) C. Gross resection of primary lesion associated with involved regional lymph nodes and microscopic residual demonstrated by involvement of the margin of resection
III	Regional disease, incomplete resection or biopsy with gross residual disease
IV	Distant metastases, present at onset (lung, liver, bone marrow, brain, and distant soft tissue and lymph node)

Staging

The staging system employed in the first two protocols of the IRS was actually a surgical-pathologic staging system rather than a true pretreatment process (see Table 13-6). The patients allocated to group I included only those with completely resected sarcomas without evidence of regional spread. For those patients assigned to group II, gross resection of their tumors was also achieved but there was either microscopic evidence of involvement of the surgical margin and/or some manifestation of regional spread, usually lymph node metastasis. Patients in group III had gross residual sarcoma at the primary site after biopsy or resection but no distant metastases, while group IV patients had evidence of distant metastasis. There was a significant difference in relapse rates for these individual stages (Fig. 13-8).

The allocation of patients to group IV (distant metastatic disease) had no relation to the surgeon's choice of operation in the initial IRS protocols, but the allocation of a patient to group I, II or III often depended on the operative decision that was made before the patient was actually entered into the study. Although some localized lesions were clearly not resectable (e.g., most patients in group III), others whose operation was only a biopsy before the initiation of nonoperative treatment might, alternatively, have had total resection of their lesion if the surgeon had elected to perform a more radical (and disabling) procedure at the time of initial diagnosis. Although useful and practical answers to therapeutic questions have been obtained using this protocol design, the initial observations from the first two protocols in the IRS concerning the optimal operative approach to childhood rhabdomyosarcoma are less than precise due to these features of postsurgical staging. Nevertheless, some observations during the course of this initial study have led to useful new guidelines regarding surgical management (20).

The facts that the choice of operative procedure did affect the surgical-pathologic staging in some instances and that additional prognostic information on the size and histologic type of the lesions was gained from the retrospective review of the initial IRS studies led to a proposed pretreatment TNM staging method for childhood rhabdomyosarcoma that is now being tested (see Table 13-7). Future investigations and comparisons will be facilitated by using both

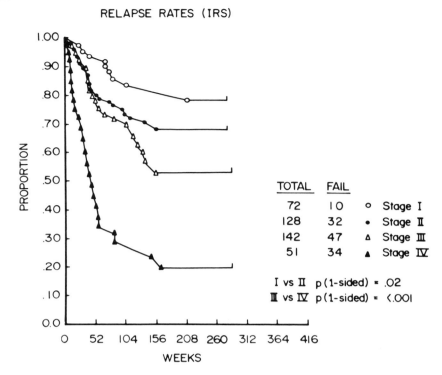

FIG. 13-8. Actuarial relapse rates in the four clinical groups of patients in IRS I.

a pretreatment staging schema and a surgical-pathologic staging process. More rigid guidelines for the operative aspects of treatment in IRS III and subsequent protocols will allow development of more precise data regarding optimal operative management, also.

Therapeutic Questions Answered by IRS I

At the onset of the IRS study for childhood rhabdomyosarcoma it had already been established that adjuvant chemotherapy played a significant role in improving disease-free and overall survival (15). The objectives of the IRS study were

1. To determine whether postoperative radiation of the tumor bed was necessary when combination chemotherapy (vincristine, actinomycin D, and cyclophosphamide) was given for two years following complete excision of a localized rhabdomyosarcoma (clinical group I).
2. To determine whether combination chemotherapy with three drugs (vincristine, actinomycin D, and cyclophosphamide) was better than two drugs (vincristine and actinomycin D) for patients with grossly resected tumors that had microscopic margin involvement, lymph node involvement, or other regional spread (clinical group II). All patients in this group received routine postoperative radiation therapy because of regional tumor spread.
3. To determine whether the combination of three-drug chemotherapy with radiation therapy could induce and maintain remission in patients with gross residual disease after surgery (clinical group III) or metastatic disease at diagnosis (group IV), and to determine whether the addition of adriamycin to this drug combination was beneficial.

Table 13-7. Pretreatment Staging Schema for Childhood Rhabdomyosarcoma (IRS III)

Tumor

(T(site)1—confined to anatomic site of origin
   a. <5 cm
   b. ≥5 cm
T(site)2—extension into and/or fixation to surrounding tissues
   a. <5 cm
   b. ≥5 cm

Histology

G1	favorable
	embryonal, sarcoma botryoides (mixed, undifferentiated)
G2	unfavorable
	alveolar (monomorphous, anaplastic)

Regional lymph nodes

N-0	no clinically involved regional nodes
N-1	clinically involved regional nodes
N-X	clinical status of regional nodes unknown (especially sites that preclude regional lymph node evaluation)

Metastasis

M-0	no distant metastasis
M-1(sites)	metastases present; subscript indicates site(s)

Subscripts for T (site)	*Subscripts for M (site)*
hn—head and neck	dn—distant nodes
or—orbit	lu—lung or positive pleural effusion
ex—extremities	li—liver
ex-lg—limb girdle	b—bone
gu—pelvic GU	m—marrow
te—paratesticular	n—CNS or positive CSF
ot—other (includes trunk, retroperitoneum, and perineum)	s—soft tissue other than nodes
	p—peritoneum or positive ascitic fluid

Summary of pretreatment clinical staging based on clinical, radiographic and laboratory examination (plus histologic biopsy):

A small, nonextensive tumor with favorable histology and clinically negative nodes

B large and/or extensive tumor with favorable histology and clinically negative lymph nodes

C any size or extent of tumor with clinically involved regional nodes and/or unfavorable histology

D distant metastasis

A T1a, G1, N0(X), M0

B T1b, 2a, 2b, G1, N0(X), M0

C T1–2, G1–2, N1, M0 or T1–2, G2, N0, M0

D any T, any G, any N, M-1

   T and M will have appropriate subscripts

It is of interest that no significant advantage was apparent from the addition of postoperative radiotherapy in the group of patients who had completely resected rhabdomyosarcomas (clinical group I) and received adjuvant chemotherapy for the two-year period (Fig. 13-9). (This finding and its implication for the treatment of adult sarcomas are discussed in Chapter 11.) In those patients with regional disease (clinical group II) who had chemotherapy and regional radiotherapy after surgery, the disease-free survival difference between the two- and three-drug regimens was not significant (Fig. 13-10).

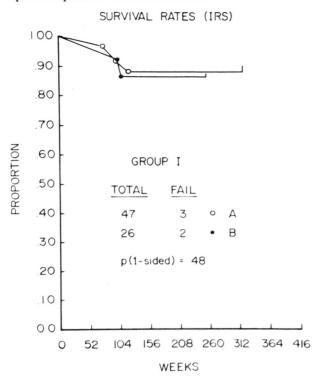

SURVIVAL RATES (IRS)

GROUP I

TOTAL	FAIL		
47	3	○	A
26	2	●	B

p(1-sided) = 48

WEEKS

FIG. 13-9. Actuarial survival rates for nonradiated (*A*) and radiated (*B*) randomized patients in clinical group I of IRS I. (All patients had complete surgical excision and VAC chemotherapy program for two years.)

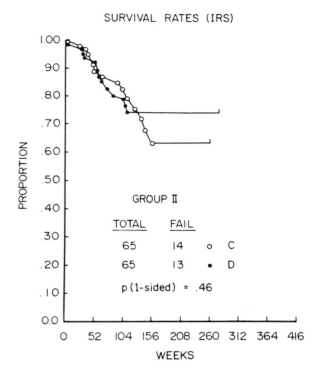

SURVIVAL RATES (IRS)

GROUP II

TOTAL	FAIL		
65	14	○	C
65	13	●	D

p(1-sided) = .46

WEEKS

FIG. 13-10. Actuarial survival curves for children in group II of IRS I on regimens consisting of VAC for two years (*D*) or a more intensive vincristine and actinomycin D regimen for one year (*C*). All patients had gross excision and postoperative local irradiation.

This finding has some practical significance, since the overall control rates in the surgically resected patient groups were high enough now to begin this examination of means of reducing the morbidity of the treatment program. A disappointing finding in the nonresected groups of patients (clinical groups III and IV) was that adriamycin did not add to the disease control rates for childhood rhabdomyosarcoma patients receiving three-drug (vincristine, actinomycin D, and cyclophosphamide) chemotherapy (Fig. 13-11). This finding was in contrast to the benefits expected on the basis of the observed effectiveness of adriamycin in adults with soft-tissue sarcomas.

Of particular importance in this overall study was the finding that *both* surgical resection and adjuvant chemotherapy are vitally important to the achievement of high disease control rates (except for the orbital lesions). The important role of radiotherapy in the control of regional disease, particularly with the orbital and parameningeal sites, was also striking. A disappointing observation was the finding that recurrence after this combined treatment program, either local or metastatic, indicated a poor prognosis no matter what the initial surgical-pathologic grouping.

Additional Observations from the Early IRS Studies (I and II)
A preponderance of patients in IRS I and II were in group III (regional nonresected sarcoma) and group IV (distant metastatic disease). Nonresectable sarcomas were more frequent in some anatomic sites (e.g., head and neck) than in others, and the designation "nonresectable" was the physician's choice in some instances (e.g., the orbit and some extremity lesions that would other-

SURVIVAL RATES (IRS)

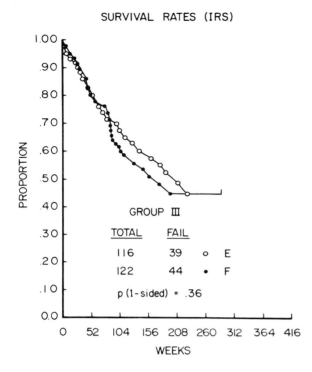

GROUP III

TOTAL	FAIL		
116	39	o	E
122	44	•	F

p (1-sided) = .36

FIG. 13-11. Actuarial survival curves for children in group III of IRS I (incomplete excision followed by irradiation and chemotherapy). There was no difference in results between the VAC regimen (E) and this same regimen with adriamycin added (F).

wise require amputation). In any event, complete resection was less frequently feasible for the total population of patients with childhood rhabdomyosarcoma than has been the case for soft-tissue sarcomas in the adult population. The data in Figure 13-8 that show the survival based on surgical-pathologic staging in IRS I clearly demonstrate that operative removal, if feasible (groups I and II), led to a better prognosis. A striking exception to this general rule was the patient group with orbital rhabdomyosarcoma, as this group did prove to have an excellent prognosis following a nonoperative (radiation and chemotherapy) program.

A second general observation from IRS I and II was the variation in prognosis associated with some differences in histopathologic classification. The histologic variants of rhabdomyosarcoma as initially defined did not seem to alter the prognosis for patients entered into this study except for those with the alveolar histology. This histologic subtype was more frequent in the perineal (69%), extremity (44%), and trunk (38%) sites than head and neck (13%), orbit (6%), and genitourinary (4%) sites. Patients with alveolar histology who had complete surgical resection of the primary lesion had a distinctly higher relapse rate (Table 13-8) than did patients with embryonal or other histologic types. This presence of a prognostically unfavorable histologic type or types may partly explain the differences in prognosis associated with lesions that arise at various anatomic sites (e.g., the extremities). In addition, it may well affect the aggressiveness of therapy in the future for patients who are selected for differing treatments depending on histologic type.

A third surprising observation related to incidence of lymphatic spread. In the past, clinicopathologic reviews of children with rhabdomyosarcoma yielded conflicting information regarding the frequency of this route of spread. A review of 264 eligible entries in the early part of IRS I revealed that lesions in the extremities (17%) and genitourinary tract (19%) were associated with a higher than expected incidence of lymphatic spread, and those of the orbit (0%), head and neck region (3%), and trunk (10%) with a lower incidence.

201

A subset of the genitourinary sites, the paratesticular region, had a 43% incidence of lymphatic spread (21). All of these were minimum figures for lymphatic spread, since the investigators made no special efforts to biopsy nonpalpable regional nodes in this earlier study. A concerted effort is now being made by planned biopsy procedures to obtain more accurate figures on the incidence of lymphatic spread and its prognostic implications.

Both the preliminary observations and ongoing evaluations of lymphatic spread should encourage the surgeon to either biopsy or dissect the regional lymph nodes in all children with rhabdomyosarcoma. For most sites, adequate regional lymph node biopsy, rather than a formal dissection, seems appropriate for nonpalpable nodes since, thus far, the data do not justify the disability incurred by a standard regional lymph node dissection as a routine part of the operation. However, a formal retroperitoneal lymph node dissection is clearly indicated for paratesticular lesions because of the incidence of metastatic nodes observed and the inaccessibility of this particular site for simple biopsy. The higher incidence of metastases and the relatively inaccessible lymph nodes relating to other pelvic genitourinary sites appear to provide an indication for formal dissection in this region also, but this may be deferred in those patients in whom nonoperative therapies are administered prior to subsequent surgical resection. Data to establish the therapeutic value of this approach are being developed, but the actual findings regarding incidence have encouraged a more aggressive approach to regional lymph nodes in children with rhabdomyosarcoma.

Observations Concerning Special Anatomic Sites

The Extremities

Approximately one-fifth of the patients with childhood rhabdomyosarcoma had lesions arising in the upper or lower extremities, while most adults with rhabdomyosarcoma (approximately 80%) have lesions arising from the extremities. One of the observations of most concern in children has been a poorer prognosis for extremity lesions than for lesions in other anatomic sites (Table 13-9) (14). This is in contrast to patients treated prior to the days of combined-modality therapy, when extremity primary sites had the best prognosis (28). Although not clearly established, the higher incidence of alveolar lesions in the extremities (32%) than in all other sites (16%) may explain this unfavorable prognosis, as this histopathologic type is associated with a higher overall relapse rate (Table 13-8). Alveolar lesions probably justify more intensive nonoperative treatment, but a more radical operation, or even amputation, is another possible means for dealing with this unfavorable group. It will be difficult to test this hypothesis directly in a randomized clinical trial, but data thus far encourage a particularly aggressive approach to this subpopulation of patients.

Table 13-8. Relapse Rates for Groups I and II by Histopathologic Type (IRS I)

Histopathology	No. of patients	No. who had relapses	Percent
Alveolar	37	17	46*
Embryonal	107	16	15*
Other	48	8	17

* p < 0.0001.

Table 13-9. Disease-Free Survival Two Years
after Initiation of Treatment (IRS I)

Lesion sites	Group I, %	Group II, %
All	83	72
Extremity	62*	63†
Genitourinary	92*	79†

* p < 0.02.
† Percentage is not significant.

Early in the study, the data from the IRS demonstrated the reluctance of many surgeons to perform truly radical resections or amputations for extremity lesions. This was based on the early enthusiasm of all surgeons for the marked benefits that were achieved by effective adjuvant chemotherapy. Actually, the few patients in IRS I who were subjected to amputation did quite poorly, but this outcome may have been due to advanced-stage tumors or to poor patient selection for this procedure (e.g., patients with unrecognized distant metastases). Improved staging with CT scans will be of great benefit in controlling this factor. The effect of determination of stage by the type of operation performed rather than solely on the clinical extent of disease is best seen in the treatment results of the early group of patients with rhabdomyosarcoma in an extremity in IRS I. Careful review of the records of 14 patients with rhabdomyosarcoma of the extremities who were classified as group III (partial excision or biopsy only) demonstrated that 10 actually had anatomic lesions that could have been resected by a more radical operation if the surgeon had not elected to rely on nonoperative therapy to achieve local control. Eleven of the initial 14 patients in group III have relapsed (78%), an extremely high failure rate compared with the relapse rate of 36% of those undergoing total gross resection of the sarcoma (groups I and II). This disparity in failure rates should encourage the surgeon to carry out gross resection of all rhabdomyosarcomas whenever possible and to consider amputation for the few patients who *cannot* otherwise be resected, rather than relying completely on nonoperative therapy. The better prognosis seen after total gross resection than after biopsy only for essentially comparable lesions is probably relevant to the treatment of rhabdomyosarcomas at other anatomic sites as well (with the exception of the orbit). Despite the great advances in the nonoperative therapy for childhood rhabdomyosarcoma, these limited observations from IRS I should lead to insistence on operative removal when feasible, either before or after the nonoperative phase of treatment.

Head and Neck Rhabdomyosarcomas

Primary lesions arising in the orbit proved to be less aggressive than those in other head and neck sites, as measured by the extent of local disease, the absence of regional lymphatic metastasis, the rarity of distant metastases, and the overall good prognosis. This high success rate for nonoperative treatment of orbital rhabdomyosarcoma was recognized before the IRS. For this reason, most orbital primary sarcomas in this study were subjected to biopsy, classified as group III lesions, and treated by nonoperative means with a high success rate (82% two-year control). The data obtained have confirmed the finding that this approach to orbital lesions gives good results and suggest that resection of lesions in this unique site is rarely required.

Another finding in the IRS was the increased hazard of local treatment failure of head and neck lesions that arise in parameningeal sites (39). On the basis of early findings in patients with lesions arising in the nasopharynx, nasal cavity, paranasal sinuses, pterygomaxillary space, and middle ear it

203

was demonstrated that there was a high risk in this group of subsequently developing direct intracranial and meningeal extension (about 35%). It was found subsequently that this local failure problem could be reduced to a large degree (about 5%) by adding radiation to the craniomeninges in continuity with the primary tumor site and adding intrathecal chemotherapy to the treatment program in selected patients (those with intracranial extension, bone erosion, and/or cranial nerve palsy) (33).

Paratesticular Lesions

Children with rhabdomyosarcoma in this site have a high incidence of lymphatic metastasis (see earlier discussion), and this has led to the recommendation that these patients should undergo routine retroperitoneal lymph node dissection (32). This dissection also proved to be a potential benefit in terms of the selection of patients for adjuvant radiotherapy, since the morbidity associated with radiotherapy to this regional lymph node basin could be avoided in patients who were found to be without lymph node metastasis (40). Another feature of the treatment of paratesticular lesions, when postoperative radiotherapy is employed, is the necessity to reduce the chance of damage to the contralateral normal testis. Temporary transposition of the remaining testis to the adjacent thigh with later replacement in the scrotum is now recommended on the assumption that, despite shielding, the remaining testis is exposed to some potential damage during radiation to the regional lymph node area. It is of interest that paratesticular lesions have an excellent prognosis (89% two-year survival) despite their high incidence of lymphatic metastasis.

Prostate, Bladder, and Vagina

Sarcomas arising from these sites, when treated by primary surgical resection, may require partial or total exenteration to achieve adequate removal. Because of the three pelvic organs in the female, it is easier than it is in males to spare the bladder in patients with posteriorly placed lesions and the rectum in those with anteriorly placed lesions.

When patients in IRS I who underwent pelvic exenteration for rhabdomyosarcoma of the bladder and received postoperative chemotherapy were compared retrospectively with those with smaller lesions who were treated by a more limited primary resection and chemotherapy, the failure rate was higher in the latter and presumably more favorable group (12). However, the control rates were still impressive, even when less aggressive surgery was employed, sometimes with inadequate margins on subsequent pathologic study. These limited retrospective observations are helpful from the standpoint of demonstrating that, when one does operate, one should remove the tumor completely, if possible, and not compromise chances for cure. It appeared from pilot data, however, that less disabling pelvic procedures might be suitable for bladder, prostate, and vaginal lesions if the nonoperative therapy was employed as the *initial* treatment rather than after surgical resection. This might allow bladder preservation, a really meaningful objective.

Although patients undergoing radical pelvic surgery combined with radiation and/or chemotherapy for bladder, prostate, or vaginal sarcomas do have an excellent prognosis, the morbidity and long-term disability associated with this method of management are primarily related to the extent of the surgical procedures, particularly when exenteration is required. Interesting observations made both in the IRS I and in pilot data from other institutions around the world concerned those patients in whom chemotherapy was used as the primary mode of therapy for various reasons unrelated to the specific protocols. This primary chemotherapeutic approach, followed in some patients by radiation and subsequent more limited but complete surgical resection, seemed to yield control rates similar to those following the more radical approach. Early analyses of studies in IRS II utilizing this concept have shown that disease-free survival figures are similar to those with the more radical approach (e.g., exenteration) (13). This initial nonoperative approach has also led to conservation of pelvic organs (particularly the bladder) in a significant proportion of patients, despite the fact that exenterative surgery is eventually required for some patients. This appears thus far to reduce the morbidity of treatment without significant sacrifice of therapeutic efficacy. From these data it appears that it may be desirable in the future to revise the general concept that chemotherapy and/or radiotherapy are adjuvants which should always follow operation. With primary chemotherapy, surgery might be considered the adjuvant therapy, although operative resection at some point in the treatment program clearly is still an important element of the multimodal management.

Summary

The IRS trials have clearly indicated that each primary site of origin of childhood rhabdomyosarcomas has special problems which affect survival and treatment programs as well. Treatment morbidity and subsequent disability are significant problems also with the more aggressive programs employed. This has led to a continuing study to evaluate the role of primary chemotherapy for special pelvic sites so as to reduce the disability from the surgery that is subsequently required. Other approaches to reduce the early and late morbidity of therapy are clearly needed for the more favorable groups at all primary sites. Meanwhile, improved protocols of therapy are required for those patients who have nonresectable and/or metastatic disease or have recurrent disease after the initial treatment program. These are the goals of current and subsequent trials.

References

1. Botting AJ, Soule EH, Brown AL: Smooth muscle tumors in children. Cancer 18:711–720, 1965.
2. Chaudhuri B, Ronan SG, Ghosh L: Benign lipoblastoma: report of a case. Cancer 46:611–614, 1980.
3. Chung FB, Enzinger FM: Infantile fibrosarcoma. Cancer 38:729–739, 1976.
4. Chung FB, Enzinger FM: Fibroma of tendon sheath. Cancer 44:1945–1954, 1979.
5. Crocker DW, Stout AP: Synovial sarcoma in children. Cancer 12:1123–1133, 1959.
6. Crussi-Gonzalez F, Wiederhold MD, Sotelo-Avila C: Congenital fibrosarcoma: presence of a histiocytic component. Cancer 46:77–86, 1980.
7. Dehner LP, Askin FB: Tumors of fibrous tissue origin in childhood: a clinicopathologic study of cutaneous and soft tissue neoplasms in 66 children. Cancer 38:888–900, 1976.
8. Enzinger FM, Winslow DJ: Liposarcoma: a study of 103 cases. Virchows Arch Path Anat 335:367–388, 1962.
9. Exelby PR, Knapper WH, Huvos AG, Beattie EJ: Soft-tissue fibrosarcoma in children. J Pediatr Surg 8:415–420, 1973.
10. Fields J, Helwig EB: Leiomyosarcoma of the skin and subcutaneous tissue. Cancer 47:156–159, 1981.
11. Hays DM, Mirabel VO, Karlan MS, Patel HR, Landing BH: Fibrosarcomas in infants and children. J Pediatr Surg 5:176–183, 1970.
12. Hays DM, Raney RB Jr, Lawrence W Jr, Soule EH, Gehan EA, Tefft M: Bladder

and prostatic tumors in the Intergroup Rhabdomyosarcoma Study (IRS I): Results of therapy. Cancer 50:1472–1482, 1982.

13. Hays DM, Raney RB Jr, Lawrence W Jr, Tefft M, Soule EH, Crist WM, Foulkes M, Maurer HM: Primary chemotherapy in the treatment of children with bladder-prostate tumors in the Intergroup Rhabdomyosarcoma Study (IRS II). J Pediatr Surg 17:812–820, 1982.

14. Hays D, Soule E, Lawrence W Jr, Gehan E, Maurer H, Donaldson M, Raney R, Tefft M: Extremity lesions in the Intergroup Rhabdomyosarcoma Study (IRS I): a preliminary report. Cancer 48:1–8, 1982.

15. Heyn RM, Holland R, Newton WA Jr, Tefft M, Breslow N, Hartman JR: The role of combined chemotherapy in the treatment of rhabdomyosarcoma in children. Cancer 34:2128–2142, 1974.

16. Jenkin D, Sonley M: Soft-tissue sarcomas in the young: medical treatment advances in perspective. Cancer 46:621–629, 1980.

17. Kauffman SL, Stout AP: Lipoblastic tumors of children. Cancer 12:912–925, 1959.

18. Kilman JW, Clatworthy HW, Newton WA, Grosfeld JL: Reasonable surgery for rhabdomyosarcoma: a study of 67 cases. Ann Surg 178:346–351, 1973.

19. Lauer DH, Enzinger FM: Cranial fasciitis of childhood. Cancer 45:401–406, 1980.

20. Lawrence W Jr, Hays DM: Surgical lessons from the Intergroup Rhabdomyosarcoma Study. J Natl Cancer Inst 56:159–163, 1981.

21. Lawrence W Jr, Hays DM, Moon TW: Lymphatic metastasis with childhood rhabdomyosarcoma. Cancer 39:556–559, 1977.

22. Lawrence W, Jegge G, Foote FW Jr: Embryonal rhabdomyosarcoma: a clinico-pathological study. Cancer 17:361–376, 1964.

23. Lee SM, Hajdu SI, Exelby PR: Synovial sarcoma in children. Surg Gynecol Obstet 138:701–704, 1974.

24. Mackenzie AR, Whitmore WF Jr, Melamed MR: Myosarcomas of the bladder and prostate. Cancer 22:833–844, 1968.

25. Maurer HM, Donaldson M, Gehan EA, Hammond D, Hays DM, Lawrence W Jr, Lindberg R, Newton W, Ragab A, Raney RB, Ruymann F, Soule EH, Sutow WW, Tefft M (for the IRS Committee): The Intergroup Rhabdomyosarcoma Study: Update—November, 1978. Natl Cancer Inst Monogr 56:61–68, 1981.

26. Neifeld JP, Berg JW, Godwin D, Salzberg AM: A retrospective epidemiologic study of pediatric fibrosarcomas. J Pediatr Surg 13:735–739, 1978.

27. Neifeld JP, Berg JW, Godwin D, Salzberg AM: A retrospective epidemiologic study of pediatric soft tissue sarcomas. Presented at the Annual Meeting of the American Academy of Pediatrics, October 1980.

28. Neifeld JP, Maurer H, Godwin D, Berg JW, Salzberg AM: Prognostic variables in pediatric rhabdomyosarcoma before and after multimodal therapy. J Pediatr Surg 14:699–703, 1979.

29. Nelson AJ III: Embryonal rhabdomyosarcoma. Report of 24 cases and study of the effectiveness of radiation therapy upon the primary tumor. Cancer 22:64–68, 1968.

30. Pack GT, Ariel IM: Sarcomas of the soft somatic tissues in infants and children. Surg Gynecol Obstet 98:675–686, 1954.

31. Pratt CB: Response of childhood rhabdomyosarcoma to combination chemotherapy. J Pediatr 74:791–794, 1969.

32. Raney RB, Hays DM, Lawrence W, Soule EH, Tefft M, Donaldson MH (for the IRS Committee): Paratesticular rhabdomyosarcoma in childhood. Cancer 42:729–736, 1978.

33. Raney RB Jr, Tefft M, Maurer HM, Newton WA, Ragab AH, Lawrence W Jr, Foulkes MA: Results of intensive treatment of children with cranial parameningeal sarcoma: a report from the Intergroup Rhabdomyosarcoma Study. Proc AACR 23:120, 1982 (abst.)

34. Sordillo PP, Helson L, Hajdu SI, Magill GB, Kosloff C, Golbey RB, Beattie EJ: Malignant schwannoma—clinical characteristics, survival, and response to therapy. Cancer 47:2503–2509, 1981.

35. Soule EH, Mahour GH, Mills SD, Lynn HB: Soft-tissue sarcomas of infants and children: a clinicopathologic study of 135 cases. Mayo Clinic Proc 43:313–326, 1968.

36. Soule EH, Pritchard DJ: Fibrosarcoma in infants and children: a review of 110 cases. Cancer 40:1711–1721, 1977.

37. Stout AP: Fibrosarcoma in infants and children. Cancer 15:1028–1040, 1962.

38. Sulamaa M, Möller C: Soft tissue sarcoma in children. J Pediatr Surg 4:520–525, 1969.

39. Tefft M, Fernandez C, Donaldson M, Newton W, Moon TE: Incidence of meningeal involvement by rhabdomyosarcoma of the head and neck in children: a report of the Intergroup Rhabdomyosarcoma Study (IRS). Cancer 42:253–258, 1978.

40. Tefft M, Hays D, Raney RB, Lawrence W, Soule E, Donaldson M, Sutow WW, Gehan E (for the IRS Committee): Radiation to regional nodes for rhabdomyosarcoma of the genitourinary tract in children: Is it necessary? A report of the Intergroup Rhabdomyosarcoma Study #1 (IRS-I). Cancer 45:3065–3068, 1980.

41. Wood DK, Das Gupta TK: Soft tissue sarcomas in infancy and childhood. J Surg Oncol 5:387–404, 1973.

42. Young JL, Miller RW: Incidence of malignant tumors in US children. J Pediatr 86:254–258, 1975.

Index